Rationing America's Medical Care

Brookings Dialogues on Public Policy

The presentations and discussions at Brookings conferences and seminars often deserve wide circulation as contributions to public understanding of issues of national importance. The Brookings Dialogues on Public Policy series is intended to make such statements and commentary available to a broad and general audience, usually in summary form. The series supplements the Institution's research publications by reflecting the contrasting, often lively, and sometimes conflicting views of elected and appointed government officials, other leaders in public and private life, and scholars. In keeping with their origin and purpose, the Dialogues are not subjected to the formal review procedures established for the Institution's research publications. Brookings publishes them in the belief that they are worthy of public consideration but does not assume responsibility for their accuracy or objectivity. And, as in all Brookings publications, the judgments, conclusions, and recommendations presented in the Dialogues should not be ascribed to the trustees, officers, or other staff members of the Brookings Institution.

Rationing America's Medical Care: The Oregon Plan and Beyond

Edited by

MARTIN A. STROSBERG

JOSHUA M. WIENER

ROBERT BAKER

with I. ALAN FEIN

THE BROOKINGS INSTITUTION / Washington, D.C.

LIBRARY OF CONGRESS CATALOG CARD NUMBER 91-077958

ISBN 0-8157-8197-0

9 8 7 6 5 4 3 2

About Brookings

The Brookings Institution is a private nonprofit organization devoted to research, education, and publication in economics, government, foreign policy, and the social sciences generally. Its principal purpose is to bring knowledge to bear on the current and emerging public policy problems facing the American people. In its research, Brookings functions as an independent analyst and critic, committed to publishing its findings for the information of the public. In its conferences and other activities, it serves as a bridge between scholarship and public policy, bringing new knowledge to the attention of decisionmakers and affording scholars a better insight into policy issues. Its activities are carried out through three research programs (Economic Studies, Governmental Studies, Foreign Policy Studies), a Center for Public Education, a Publications Program, and a Social Science Computation Center.

The Institution was incorporated in 1927 to merge the Institute for Government Research, founded in 1916 as the first private organization devoted to public policy issues at the national level; the Institute of Economics, established in 1922 to study economic problems; and the Robert Brookings Graduate School of Economics and Government, organized in 1924 as a pioneering experiment in training for public service. The consolidated institution was named in honor of Robert Somers Brookings (1850–1932), a St. Louis businessman whose leadership shaped the earlier organizations.

Brookings is financed largely by endowment and by the support of philanthropic foundations, corporations, and private individuals. Its funds are devoted to carrying out its own research and educational activities. It also undertakes some unclassified government contract studies, reserving the right to publish its findings.

A Board of Trustees is responsible for general supervision of the Institution, approval of fields of investigation, and safeguarding the independence of the Institution's work. The President is the chief administrative officer, responsible for formulating and coordinating policies, recommending projects, approving publications, and selecting staff.

v

Editors' Preface

As Americans struggle to address the dual problems of securing access to health care for the uninsured and of exploding medical care costs, the discussion of health care rationing has moved to the center of the public policy debate. A notable example is the intense public discussion that surrounds the proposal by the state of Oregon to provide universal health care while explicitly rationing which diagnoses and treatments will be covered.

The papers in this volume, which were originally presented at a conference at the Brookings Institution on May 20, 1991, advance the debate on health care rationing in many ways. Focusing largely, but not exclusively, on the Oregon proposal, they examine a wide range of ethical, methodological, legal, and political issues that must be addressed by any serious program of health care reform.

We acknowledge with thanks the financial support of the conference by Union College, Albany Medical College of Union University, Pfizer/Roerig, Glaxo, Inc., and Eli Lilly and Co. We also wish to thank Warren I. Cikins and Pamela F. Buckles of the Brookings Center for Public Policy Education and Carolyn J. Hill of the Economic Studies program for their excellent assistance in organizing the conference. We are also grateful to Rhonda Sheehan and Marianne Snowden of Union College and Barbara Sander of Albany Medical College and to Union College students Jonathan Bynum, Andrew Lippman, Julie Walter, John Whitaker, and Angelique Wolf. Carolyn Hill and Diane Maranis provided staff assistance; Carol Clark and Caroline Lalire edited the manuscript; and Susan Woollen prepared it for typesetting.

The views expressed in this volume are those of the authors and should not be ascribed to the institutions or persons acknowledged or to the trustees, officers, or staff members of the Brookings Institution.

Martin A. Strosberg
Joshua M. Wiener
Robert Baker
with I. Alan Fein

January 1992
Washington, D.C.

Contents

Introduction and Summary

Policy Questions

The Political Perspective

Physician Perspectives

Legal and Philosophical Reflections

Rationing America's Medical Care

Introduction and Summary

Introduction

"Politicians make choices in ways that will minimize and, if possible, eliminate any public perception that they are rationing care or diminishing its quality."[1] Representative Willis Gradison of the House Ways and Means Subcommittee on Health made this assessment at a 1986 Brookings conference on rationing health care for the critically ill. Only five years later, at another Brookings conference, policymakers, analysts, and health care providers met to consider a proposal that would place politicians and public institutions squarely at the center of an explicit health care rationing plan. The conference, entitled Rationing America's Medical Care: Opening Pandora's Box?, highlighted the Oregon Basic Health Services Program (hereafter the Oregon Plan). If implemented, this plan would forge a chain of accountability from clinical decisionmaking at the bedside directly to the Oregon State Legislature. This volume presents the papers from the conference of May 20, 1991.

The intent of the Oregon Plan is to address simultaneously health care for the uninsured and rising health care costs. The plan expands medicaid and private insurance to large numbers of people who currently have no health insurance, but at the price of explicitly deciding not to cover some medical procedures widely accepted as beneficial.

In brief, the Oregon Plan would do the following:

—Extend medicaid eligibility to all persons with incomes below the federal poverty level ($928 per month for a family of three in 1991) without regard to "welfare category"—that is, age, family status, pregnancy status, or employment status. The income eligibility limit for medicaid in Oregon is currently 50 percent of the federal poverty level.

—Establish a public process for defining a basic health care package for medicaid eligibles. To this end, a publicly appointed Oregon Health Services Commission has prepared a list of 709 paired medical conditions and treatments ranked according to clinical effectiveness and social importance. Integral to the priority status is the incorporation of quality-of-life measurements. The priority list was submitted to the state legislature, which, through its allocation of funds to the medicaid budget, has determined how many services on this list can be funded. Those that are too far down the list are not provided in the basic medical plan, though they might be beneficial services. In July 1991 the legislature allocated funds that covered services down to number 587 on the priority list. Examples of conditions-treatments that are near the bottom of the list are conditions that might improve spontaneously (such as viral sore throat), conditions for which a "home" treatment is effective (for example, sprains), and conditions for which treatment is either not generally effective or futile (such as surgery for low back pain and aggressive medical treatment for end-stage cancer and AIDS, and for extremely premature babies). The legislative allocation will provide medicaid eligibility to another 120,000 Oregonians, in addition to the 205,000 currently covered.

—Mandate, by 1995, universal employer health care coverage of employees and dependents with a benefit package that is equal to or greater than the one provided to the medicaid group. Many of the "near-poor" who have incomes above the federal poverty level would be helped by this coverage.

—Establish an insurance pool for "medically uninsurables"—those who do not qualify for medicaid and cannot obtain health insurance because of preexisting medical conditions.

—Create a "liability shield" that protects providers against criminal prosecution, civil liability, or professional disciplinary action when they do not provide those services that the legislature has chosen not to fund.

By far the most controversial component of the Oregon Plan is its explicit rationing, which fails to cover services at the lower end of the priority list. Yet, most of the panelists at the Brookings conference agreed that, whether by conscious choice or not, health care is already rationed in the United States for both the uninsured and the medicaid populations. In times of budgetary pressure, a typical response by state government is to reduce medicaid reimbursement to providers or to drop coverage to a portion of poor persons already on the medicaid rolls, rather than to raise taxes or draw funds from other social programs. Such responses ultimately ration care to anonymous people; government need not confront individuals. With a commitment to universal access to a basic level of health services through medicaid expansion, employer mandates, and an uninsurables pool, the debate in Oregon focuses on the services themselves, their effectiveness, and their value to the community. The debate shifts from whom to cover to what to cover, and is based on the degree to which health services improve health status. The debate was structured as an open process with a fair amount of public input. Although most of the input has been from the upper-middle class, Oregon has done a better job than most states in soliciting community values and preferences.

Many Oregonians, including Jean Thorne, Oregon's medicaid director, see their plan as a pragmatic response to a beleaguered state medicaid budget, burdened by a sinking state economy and by new federal mandates. To many others across the nation, the package of bills that embodies the Oregon Basic Health Services Act is seen not only as a bold and innovative reform of the medicaid system but as a potential model for more sweeping reform and as an alternative to federal policymaking, which is paralyzed by budget deficits.

Because medicaid is a joint federal-state program, Oregon requires the permission of Congress or the U.S. Health Care Financing Administration in the form of federal waivers of existing medicaid requirements. It is far from certain that the federal government will allow Oregon to make what many consider to be radical changes in medicaid. But it is clear that the Oregon Plan, having been placed under the national microscope, has generated a national debate over the moral, legal, political, and methodological aspects of its rationing plan.

CRITICISMS AND CHALLENGES

Although there has been a variety of challenges to the Oregon Plan, three criticisms stand out:

1. *There are alternatives to rationing. Before considering rationing, first eliminate administrative waste and nonbeneficial services.* In his remarks, Representative Bernard Sanders (Independent of Vermont) proposed a Canadian-style national health insurance system as an alternative to the Oregon Plan. In contrast to the complexity and fragmentation of the U.S. reimbursement system, the Canadian system relies on pro-

vincially controlled, single-payer health plans for reimbursement of hospitals and physicians. A frequently cited advantage of the Canadian model is that it has eliminated many of the administrative costs of multiple insurance coverages in hospitals, physicians' offices, and nursing homes. Using the research of Steffie Woolhandler and David Himmelstein, Sanders argues that if the United States can achieve the same level of administrative efficiency as Canada, it could provide 20 percent more services at the current level of funding, which would eliminate the need to ration care.[2] The Canadian model that Sanders prefers provides universal access to the same set of services regardless of income. This system prohibits selling insurance that provides benefits already covered under the provincial plans.

Short of restructuring the American health insurance industry, some claim that to contain escalating cost and to achieve a more efficient system, we need only try harder with our existing regulatory and market strategies. There has also been a renewed nationwide emphasis on identifying and eliminating from coverage nonbeneficial and inappropriately delivered services.

Can the elimination of administrative waste and nonbeneficial services (under the Oregon Plan, nonbeneficial services fall to the bottom of the list) postpone rationing indefinitely? Although providers, politicians, and consumer groups may take refuge in an affirmative answer, panelist Henry Aaron of Brookings notes that once the "one-time saving" of administrative efficiency has been achieved, the inexorable diffusion of new technologies, the aging of the population, and changing consumer tastes will increase the proportion of gross national product spent on health expenditures and lead to a renewed call for rationing. Moreover, as Robert Baker of Union College and Joshua Wiener of Brookings note, the Canadian and European systems of universal coverage ration care by limiting the availability of high-technology services.

2. *The prioritization process and the resultant list are flawed morally and methodologically.* The list and the process that generated it have been intensely scrutinized. The papers by Michael Garland and Robert Kaplan describe the process: the discovery of community values and the incorporation of these values into a scheme that considers the comparative benefits that each service would bring to the entire population. Michael Garland is cofounder and former president of Oregon Health Decisions, a grass-roots citizen forum that helped to facil-

itate public involvement in setting priorities. Robert Kaplan is the developer of the quality-of-well-being (QWB) scale that was used as a basis for incorporating quality-of-life assessments into the definition of health care benefit. He is also a proponent of cost-utility analysis as a method for determining appropriate resource allocation, which is based on the principle of producing the greatest benefit for the most people.

Of considerable concern to the Oregon Health Services Commission and to those closely observing the proceedings was the question of where highly beneficial but also very expensive services would rank on the priority list. In a traditional cost-utility analysis, a highly beneficial life-sustaining service could be outweighed by its high cost or by the fact that only a few people will benefit, and so be driven toward the bottom of the list.[3] In May 1990, using conventional cost-utility principles, the Health Services Commission generated an initial list in which this phenomenon appeared. For example, a procedure for capping teeth received a higher priority than an appendectomy, a ranking that struck the commissioners as counterintuitive and provoked widespread public criticism.

In response, in February 1991 the commission generated a new list, using an "alternative methodology." Departing from a strict use of cost-utility principles, this alternative methodology allowed the commissioners to organize the list of 709 conditions-treatments according to seventeen different categories (for example, acute fatal conditions for which treatment allows full recovery, prevention care for children, comfort care) that reflected community values. They were also able to adjust the list by moving certain life-saving services to a higher, and intuitively more sensible, ranking. Kaplan, critical of this departure, argues that a more rigorous and sustained analysis, using better information on treatment effectiveness, would have generated an initial list with rankings less counterintuitive and more likely to produce an allocation providing greater benefit to more people.

The ranking system and the list itself are intended to be refined over time. Nevertheless, they have been criticized on moral as well as on methodological grounds. John La Puma, practicing physician and bioethicist, strenuously objects to the incorporation of community-wide quality-of-life assessments of benefits into the ranking process. He warns that the collectively determined values and preferences may differ significantly from those of the individual patient. And it is the responsibility of the physician to individualize treatment based on the patient's preferences. Furthermore, La Puma questions how a physician can ethically participate in a publicly sanctioned, two-tiered system, with medicaid patients receiving fewer benefits than nonmedicaid patients.

Robert Veatch of Georgetown University, in contrast, argues that in a world of finite resources, including medicaid budgets, it is morally irresponsible not to ration marginally beneficial services. He finds the public quantification of pain, suffering, and the value of life to be preferable to the vague and subjective process that inevitably takes place at the bedside.

Above and beyond the discussion of the ethics of the prioritization process, Aaron points out the sheer complexity, and what he considers the folly, of collapsing more than 10,000 medical diagnoses into 709 pairs of medical conditions and treatments. Both Aaron and Veatch emphasize that the patients falling within these 709 categories are not uniform with respect to severity of illness, prognosis, or marginal benefit to be derived from treatment. Although he has reservations about the methodology, Veatch still believes that the Oregon Plan is a step in the right direction. Aaron, however, who is also convinced that sustained, long-term reductions in the growth of health care spending will occur only if we are willing to ration, believes the Oregon methodology is hopelessly flawed and will self-destruct in reaction to "horror" stories of patients not receiving "obviously needed" services.

To understand the centrality of Oregon's priority setting to the concept of explicit rationing, consider other national health systems like the British National Health Service. In this system, as Wiener points out, the supply of resources—number of beds and pieces of equipment—is fixed as a matter of public policy. Physicians prioritize access—ration—within the societally determined resource constraints. Of course, in the United States, there is "supply-side" rationing as well. William Shoemaker, chief of emergency medicine at the Martin Luther King Hospital in the Watts section of Los Angeles, points out that the immediate needs of patients in life-threatening conditions frequently overwhelm the capabilities of inner-city emergency rooms and critical care units.

American physicians do not necessarily shun the role of rationer. Increasingly, in health maintenance organizations, physicians are thought of as gatekeepers to resources that are limited by a fixed budget. Stephen Ayres and Anthony Tartaglia, both medical educators, call for an enhanced role for primary care physicians as gatekeepers. Ayres further argues that the primary care or personal physician, as opposed to an impersonal process, is in the best position to balance the benefits, risks, burdens, and costs of treatment.

In Oregon it is the demand that would be rationed according to explicit criteria; the services are already in existence. How much more difficult, then, will it be to deny beneficial services to a person with a condition that falls below the publicly announced cutoff point, especially while others may be receiving these services!

3. *It is unfair to single out the medicaid population to bear the brunt of rationing.* Although the Oregon Plan will improve access to health care for poor people on average, and perhaps achieve higher aggregate health status, it is the current medicaid recipients who will be asked to forgo certain beneficial services to help make some of these improvements possible. Sara Rosenbaum of the Children's Defense Fund opposes making poor children involuntarily participate in an experiment that includes substantial risks. Furthermore, she points out the inconsistency of the Oregon Plan with the objectives of the early and periodic screening, diagnosis, and treatment program (EPSDT) designed to assure medicaid children access to expanded benefits for a broad range of primary and preventive services. Recent congressional amendments to the EPSDT program prohibit limitations of these services based on considerations other than medical necessity.

Norman Daniels raises an additional question: is it fair to single out vulnerable groups like poor women and children when higher-income groups are not asked to make equivalent sacrifices? Daniels, a philosopher, and others differentiate between moral principles and political tactics. The force of the moral criticism is diminished if one believes the Oregon Plan is the first incremental step toward a single-tiered health care system that will require equal sacrifice across social classes. Political judgment naturally is considered in balancing the likelihood of the passage of comprehensive national health care reform legislation against the increasingly intolerable conditions of the status quo. Those who believe that a more comprehensive reform is currently politically infeasible tend to view opposition to incremental reform such as the Oregon Plan as tantamount to favoring the status quo.

Representative Ron Wyden (Democrat of Oregon), a member of the influential Subcommittee on Health and Environment of the House Energy and Commerce Committee, is a supporter of the Oregon Plan. Wyden, on the liberal wing of the political spectrum, regards the plan as a way to expand access and bring more resources into the system, and as a potential step toward a universal, single-tiered system. H. Tristram Engelhardt and E. Haavi Morreim, however, also supporters of the Oregon Plan, view the public construction of the basic health care plan as the legitimization of a multitiered system. Their papers outline the legal, moral, and economic foundations of a market-driven, multitiered system.

In counterpoint to Representative Sanders and other proponents of an egalitarian, single-tiered system, Engelhardt, a professor of medicine and philosophy, argues that the market and a multitiered system need no moral apology. Only the market, and not a particular vision of justice, fairness, or the common good, can give expression to the diversity of human values with regard to health care. Consistent with the President's Commission for the Study of Ethical Problems in Medicine, Engelhardt calls for an adequate level of care for all citizens, but does not deny to others the option of purchasing services above the adequate level. Oregon, through its public processes, has now defined the adequate minimum standard of care.

THE OREGON PLAN AND BEYOND

The United States, which has the highest per capita health care costs in the world, has failed to guarantee health insurance to all its citizens. Because of an escalation of these twin problems, the discussion of explicit health care rationing in the United States has gained new prominence.

It is in this context that the Oregon Plan has become the centerpiece for the serious debate about whether health care rationing is desirable and, if so, how it should be handled. As a concrete proposal, it has crystallized many of the issues that must be confronted in any major effort to reform the American health care system. Questions such as: Who will be covered? What services will be reimbursed? If not all services are covered, what criteria will be used to decide which services will not be covered? What role will community and patient values and preferences play in coverage decisions? To what extent will high technology be covered? Do the poor and nonpoor have equal access to the same set of services? Who will bear the burden of financing care to the uninsured and of containing costs? Whether the Oregon Plan is ever approved or adopted, the issues the proposal raises will be part of the public policy debate for a long time to come.

NOTES

1. Willis D. Gradison, Jr., "Federal Policy and Intensive Care," in *Rationing of Medical Care for the Critically Ill*, ed. Martin A. Strosberg, I. Alan Fein, and James D. Carroll (Brookings, 1989), p. 37.

2. Steffie Woolhandler and David U. Himmelstein, "The Deteriorating Administrative Efficiency of the U.S. Health Care System," *New England Journal of Medicine*, vol. 324 (May 2, 1991), pp. 1243–58.

3. David C. Hadorn, "Setting Health Care Priorities in Oregon: Cost-effectiveness Meets the Rule of Rescue," *Journal of the American Medical Association*, vol. 265 (May 1, 1991), pp. 2218–25.

JOSHUA M. WIENER

Rationing in America: Overt and Covert

Interest in health care rationing has exploded over the last five years. No longer solely the province of a few medical ethicists and other academics, it has moved to the center of the health policy debate as a serious option for cost containment and as a possibly necessary precondition of providing health care to the uninsured. For example, the state of Oregon proposes covering all poor people under its medicaid program but would eliminate coverage of some medical procedures widely accepted as beneficial.[1] Health insurers and benefit managers for large corporations are increasingly being asked by patients and providers to decide whether certain very expensive, but potentially lifesaving, medical treatments will be reimbursed.[2] Concern about rationing is reflected in the medicare program in such policy questions as whether medicare should pay for liver transplants or, more broadly, whether the Health Care Financing Administration should use cost factors in determining whether to cover new procedures and devices.[3]

WHAT DOES HEALTH CARE RATIONING MEAN?

No country provides completely unlimited health care resources to all its citizens. Rationing, mostly in the form of limiting services by ability to pay, is already widely practiced in the United States.[4] For example, among persons in poor or fair health, the uninsured have only half as many physician visits as the insured do.[5] Within the health care service system, recent studies suggest, people receive different treatment depending on their insurance status.[6] Despite the fact that end-stage renal disease is more common among racial minorities than among whites, fewer blacks than whites undergo kidney transplants.[7] Moreover, medicare did not cover liver transplants until recently and still does not cover prescription drugs or long-term care; access to these services is largely determined by ability to pay.

As widespread as this rationing is, it is largely the unintended result of other decisions about the health care system. Thus, the low rate of physician use by the uninsured is the consequence of the choices Americans have made about how health insurance should be distributed. It is not the result of a conscious decision that certain persons should receive limited access to medical care.

For most people with medicare, medicaid, and private insurance, however, cost is not currently an important component of treatment decisions. Doctors order whatever tests and procedures they think are medically desirable, and third parties pay for whatever the doctor deems appropriate. Ethical standards for physicians emphasize their role as patient advocates who must do whatever is medically possible to help prolong the life of the patient.[8] Rationing here means failing to provide some medical services that would be clinically beneficial. What is new in the debate is that people are beginning to talk about rationing for the insured as well as for the uninsured. Moreover, rationing is being discussed as an explicit, rather than implicit, policy choice.

WHY THE INTEREST IN RATIONING?

The new interest in health care rationing is the result of the extremely high rate of increase in health care expenditures combined with the perception that other efforts at cost containment have failed. National health expenditures increased from $249 billion in 1980 to $671 billion in 1990—an annual rate of increase of 10.4 percent.[9] As a share of the gross national product, health care increased from 9.1 percent in 1980 to 12.2 percent in 1990 and shows no signs of leveling off. Similarly, medicare expenditures increased from $32.1 billion in 1980 to $98.1 billion in 1990, an annual rate of increase of 11.8 percent.[10] Large employers saw their health insurance premiums increase by an average of 37 percent between 1988 and 1990.[11] These high rates of increase for health expenditures are largely attributable to the interaction of third-party reimbursement, which reduces cost-conscious behavior, and a technological imperative that leads medicine toward ever more expensive services.[12]

In itself, an increase in health care expenditures need not be a matter of concern. A similar increase in spending for domestically manufactured computers would be cause for cheers, not handwringing. The problem derives from the widespread perception that Americans are spending much more on medical care but not getting much healthier. In the jargon of economists, the worry is that the marginal benefit of additional spending is not worth the marginal cost. Moreover, there is increasing fear that high costs will make health insurance unaffordable for a growing number of Americans.

This anxiety about whether we are getting our money's worth has combined with the perception that health care costs are completely out of control. Governments and employers have largely done what health care experts in the early 1980s told them to do to control costs.[13] Although it is important not to overstate the extent to which changes have actually been implemented, governments and employers have introduced prospective payment, raised deductibles and coinsurance, developed preferred provider organizations, encouraged enrollment in health maintenance organizations, and imposed managed care through utilization review, second opinion programs, and prior authorization requirements. All these efforts were intended to reduce inappropriate use, improve efficiency, and control the income of providers without reducing medically beneficial services. Despite these changes, the rate of increase in health care spending has not substantially declined.[14] Rightly or wrongly, it is widely perceived that our bag of tricks for cost containment is fairly empty. As a result, there is a sense of desperation about controlling health care costs that did not previously exist.

MUST WE CHOOSE BETWEEN SERVICES FOR THE ELDERLY AND HEALTH CARE FOR THE UNINSURED?

Much of the current policy debate about health care rationing implicitly assumes that a direct trade-off exists between providing high-technology services to the elderly and providing basic health care for the uninsured. Proponents of this view contend that the United States is spending too much on the elderly and not enough on the nonelderly, especially children. There is little evidence, however, that cuts in high-technology services for the elderly will automatically translate into increased funding for programs for the uninsured. Social insurance programs for the elderly and welfare programs for adults and children have very different political dynamics and constituencies. Political support for services for the elderly is very strong and widespread. According to a public opinion survey by the Northwestern National Life Insurance Company, 65 percent of Americans oppose cutting health services to the elderly as a way of financing services for children.[15] Conversely, there is not much evidence that increasing spending for the uninsured will mean less money for high-technology health services.

These trade-offs do not exist, because the United States does not have a fixed budget for either the medicare and medicaid programs or overall national health spending.[16] Thus, it is impossible to say where the money "saved" from constraints in health spending would go. In countries that have a socially determined health budget, cuts in one area can be justified on the grounds that the money will be spent on other, higher-priority services. This closed system of funding provides a moral underpinning for resource allocation across a range of potentially unlimited demands. In the United States, it is difficult to refuse additional resources for patients, because there is no certainty that the funds will be put to better use elsewhere.

In addition, although rationing is often proposed as a way to provide everyone a "basic" level of health care, the definition of this level of care is extremely contentious.[17] Insofar as basic care means third-party payment for low-technology medicine, it is unclear why coverage for these services is morally preferable to coverage for high-technology services, such as liver transplants, which can often mean the difference between life and death. To be sure, the person may still die after receiving the high-technology service, but most of us do not face that prospect when we go to the doctor. Conversely, if basic care is so broadly defined as to include unlimited access to high-technology services, it is unclear how health care costs will ever be either controlled or made more affordable.

It is in this context that Oregon has made a real contribution by offering a specific definition of what it considers to be basic care and by recasting some of the arguments over high- and low-technology health sevices. The Oregon priority list finesses some of this debate by giving relatively high priority both to some highly valued low-technology services such as prenatal care and to some costly, but potentially life-saving, high-technology services such as kidney transplants. Lower rankings are assigned services that are not as likely to involve life-or-death issues or that are less likely to be successful.

DO OTHER COUNTRIES RATION?

As Americans seek solutions to the problems of health care costs and care for the uninsured, they have shown increasing interest in the health care systems of Canada and other industrialized countries. These countries are particularly interesting because they refute the traditional American arguments about the relationship between health care costs and the uninsured. The usual American argument is that we cannot afford to cover the uninsured because it will cost too much and will further exacerbate cost-increasing pressures in the health system. In contrast, the other countries essentially contend that the only way to control health care costs is to cover everyone and thereby control the entire health care system.

Other Western industrialized countries spend less per capita on health care than the United States does. For example, in 1989 per capita health care expenditures in the United States were $2,354, but only $1,683 in Canada, $1,274 in France, $1,232 in Germany, $1,050 in Italy, $1,035 in Japan, and $836 in the United Kingdom.[18] In general, other countries have lower per capita costs because of lower health care prices, lower administrative costs, and less availability of high-technology services.

The degree to which medical technology is constrained varies widely across countries and services, but undoubtedly privately insured Americans have greater access to many high-technology services. For example, the United States has twice the rate per million persons receiving treatment for end-stage renal disease than Great Britain has.[19] The United States has more than twice as many open heart surgical units per million persons as Canada and nearly five times as many as West Germany.[20] Similarly, the United States has four times as many magnetic resonance imagers per million persons as West Germany and seven times as many as Canada.[21] This variation is due partly to a lack of money for equipment and partly to a more skeptical view of technology on the part of physicians in other countries.[22]

Although the easy availability of high technology in the United States is good news for patients who have insurance that covers these services, it is a mixed blessing in many ways, both because of the higher costs they generate and because some of the technology is inappropriately applied. Mark Chassin and others suggest that perhaps 17 percent of coronary angiographies, 32 percent of carotid endarectomies, and 17 percent of upper gastrointestinal endoscopies performed were inappropriate.[23] Similarly, Constance Winslow and others found that 14 percent of coronary artery bypasses and 20 percent of pacemaker implants were inappropriate.[24] Although these studies are highly controversial, most people in the health policy community believe that there is more art than science in much of the practice of medicine and that new technologies are often adopted without a good sense of which patients can be expected to benefit and by how much.[25]

WOULD RATIONING CONTROL COSTS?

Although the answer to this question might obviously seem to be "yes," a more useful answer is that "it depends." First, as mentioned, every other country's health care per capita spending is only a fraction of what is spent in the United States. But once that level of health care is established, there do not appear to be huge differences in the rate of increase in expenditures due exclusively to health care factors, although most countries do have a lower rate of increase. For example, between 1975 and 1987, there was only about a 1.7 percentage point difference between the United States and the United Kingdom in the rate of increase in health care expenditures due to health care inflation in excess of general inflation and increases in medical care use (such as physician visits per person).[26] Similarly, the rate of increase in the United States was only 0.7 percentage point higher than in Canada, 0.9 percentage point higher than in France, and 1.9 percentage point higher than in Germany.[27] Health care expenditures in Japan actually increased 0.6 percentage point per year faster than in the United States.[28] These differences in the rate of increase are significant, especially when compounded over long periods of time, but they are not enormous. Although the extent to which services are rationed in these other countries is debatable, there is undoubtedly more rationing of high-technology services than in the United States, and the United Kingdom represents an extreme that would be politically intolerable in this country.

Second, some of the proposed schemes limit the rationing to the elderly population, particularly the population over age 75 or 80.[29] In a provocative study of elderly decedents, however, Anne Scitovsky found that high-cost medical services may already be allocated according to some sense of ultimate result.[30] Decedents who were in poor functional condition at the time of the fatal illness received far less in the way of physician and hospital services than did those in good functional condition. In other words, some rationing is already taking place.

Similarly, much is often made of the fact that 28 percent of medicare expenditures are provided in the last year of life.[31] But prognosis is often difficult to determine. Studies of the outcomes of critical care show that costs are highest in those cases in which the outcome was inaccurately predicted—for example, people who were supposed to die quickly and did not, and people who were supposed to get better and did not.[32]

Moreover, as William Schwartz and Henry Aaron have shown, rationing that is applied only to the population aged 75 and over cannot significantly change the rate of increase in national health expenditures.[33] Although people aged 75 and older have three times the per capita acute care health expenditures of people under age 75, they are not that numerous.[34] In 1988 the United States had 12.5 million people aged 75 and over and 233.9 million people under age 75.[35] As a result, the very elderly account for about 15 percent of acute care expenditures. Thus, even if physician and hospital services to this age group were cut by a third, it would not dramatically change either the level of health care expenditures or their rate of increase.

Conversely, rationing schemes that focus exclusively on the non-elderly population, such as Oregon's plan, are troubling because they exclude the population most willing to accept—indeed, to want—less-than-heroic efforts to prolong life. Although the right-to-die movement must be distinguished from proposals for health care rationing, both raise questions about when it is no longer appropriate to provide aggressive medical treatment.[36]

Third, people often presume that if expensive, high-technology procedures, such as organ transplants, are not provided, all the money associated with these procedures will be saved. That is not likely to happen, because these patients will continue to receive more conventional services in lieu of the high-technology alternative. In a study comparing the treatment costs of leukemia, Gilbert Welch and Eric Larson found that the costs of conventional chemotherapy were 70 percent of the costs of bone marrow transplants.[37]

Finally, one must understand that service rationing in other countries is approached much differently from the way often proposed in this country, such as in the Oregon medicaid plan. In the United Kingdom, for example, resources are limited and are allocated subject to that constraint. In other words, the British have supply-side rationing. Even though the elderly are much less likely to receive renal dialysis in the United Kingdom than in the United States, there is no official policy of denying care. Rather, as Aaron and Schwartz found, the United Kingdom limits the number of dialysis machines and the availability of staff to run them.[38] General practitioners are relied on to deflect elderly patients from dialysis so as to keep them from overloading the system.

By contrast, the American health care system begins with excess hospital capacity and numerous physicians who are specialists eager to practice their craft. Thus, the medical care system has the physical capacity to perform almost any procedure imaginable, including those that the political system may consciously choose not to cover. Explicit or demand-side rationing in this environment will be susceptible to a great many poignant personal appeals for coverage and will be extremely difficult to sustain politically.

MUST WE EXPLICITLY RATION HEALTH CARE?

The answer to the question whether explicit rationing should be introduced in the United States depends in part on people's tolerance of increased health care expenditures and in part on whether health care costs can be controlled without rationing. There is nothing magic about 11–13 percent of the gross national product that says the world will collapse if we spend more than that. Indeed, a strong argument can be made that money spent on health care is morally preferable to some alternative uses, such as expensive cars, designer clothes, and fancy jewelry. At the rate of increase in health care as a proportion of the GNP that we experienced during the 1980s, it will be nearly another twenty years before America hits 20 percent of its GNP for health care. A lot can happen during that time, and few things in life continue to increase exponentially forever. Thus, the rate of increase in health care expenditures may level off, although I would be hard pressed to say why or when this would happen of its own accord.

The second component of the answer depends on whether there are alternative ways to control health care costs. As an empirical matter, it is not true that the United States has tried all other possible methods of cost containment on a wide-scale basis. Possible alternative methods of cost containment include using single-payer rate-setting systems, reducing physician fees, eliminating unnecessary administrative costs, rooting out inappropriate utilization, and increasing enrollment in managed care.[39] Some will argue that none of these strategies will work and they may be correct, but we will not know until we try. It is troubling to ration medically effective procedures before we have truly exhausted other routes to cost containment.

CONCLUSION

Interest in health care rationing has increased greatly in recent years, largely because of the perception that alternative approaches to cost containment have failed. Although some rationing has always existed in the United States, new proposals in the policy debate explicitly suggest withholding some potentially medically effective services to the privately insured, medicare, and medicaid populations.

Whether the United States should explicitly ration health care partly depends on judgments of the likelihood of future uncontrolled increases in health care expenditures. Although the United States obviously cannot devote all its gross national product to health care, it could nevertheless continue to spend much more than it does now. Similarly, although it is certainly true that the cost-containment record of the last decade has been dismal, many possible reforms have not been widely implemented.

Finally, although rationing is sometimes presented as a panacea to the health care cost problem, the reality is more complicated. While countries differ greatly in their per capita health care costs, they differ much less in the rate of increase in health expenditures because of health care inflation and utilization. Once a country has chosen its "style" of medical care, it seems to face cost-increasing pressures that are similar across countries. Moreover, mounting evidence shows that a fair amount of rationing is already occurring in the American system, if by that one means resource allocation by expected final outcome. Thus, additional savings may be especially painful to achieve.

NOTES

1. John Kitzhaber, "A Healthier Approach to Health Care," *Issues in Science and Technology*, vol. 7 (Winter 1990–91), pp. 59–65; and Jean Thorne, "The Oregon Plan: Rejecting Invisible Rationing," *The Internist*, July–August 1990, pp. 9–11.

2. Glenn Kramon, "Rockwell's Point Man in the Health-Care Campaign," *New York Times*, April 7, 1991, p. 5D.

3. Carl Irwin, testimony presented at "Organ Transplants: Choices and Criteria, Who Lives, Who Dies, Who Pays?" Hearing of the House Select Committee on Aging, Washington, April 26, 1991; Robert E. Wren, statement presented at ibid.; and Robert Pear, "Medicare to Weigh Cost as a Factor in Reimbursement," *New York Times*, April 21, 1991, p. A1.

4. Jeffrey C. Merrill and Alan B. Cohen, "The Emperor's New Clothes: Unraveling the Myths about Rationing," *Inquiry*, vol. 24 (Summer 1987), pp. 105–09.

5. Howard E. Freeman and others, "Uninsured Working-Age Adults: Characteristics and Consequences," *Health Services Research*, vol. 24 (February 1990), p. 819.

6. Mark B. Wenneker, Joel S. Weissman, and Arnold M. Epstein, "The Association of Payer with Utilization of Cardiac Procedures in Massachusetts," *Journal of the American Medical Association*, vol. 264 (September 12, 1990), pp. 1255–95; and Jack Hadley, Earl P. Steinberg, and Judith Feder, "Comparison of Uninsured and Privately Insured Hospital Patients," *Journal of the American Medical Association*, vol. 265 (January 16, 1991), pp. 374–79.

7. Bertram L. Kasiske and others, "The Effect of Race on Access and Outcome in Transplantation," *New England Journal of Medicine*, vol. 324 (January 31, 1991), pp. 302–07.

8. Norman Daniels, "Why Saying No to Patients in the United States Is So Hard," *New England Journal of Medicine*, vol. 314 (May 22, 1986), pp. 1380–83.

9. Author's calculations based on Malcolm Gladwell, "Health Costs' Share of GNP Up Sharply," *Washington Post*, April 23, 1991, p. A5; and Katherine R. Levitt and others, "National Health Care Spending, 1989," *Health Affairs*, vol. 10 (Spring 1991), pp. 117–30.

10. *Budget of the United States Government, Fiscal Year 1991*, pt. 7., table 43, pp. 43–44.

11. Frank Swoboda, "Health Care Costs Climb 21.6% in '90," *Washington Post*, January 29, 1991, p. D1.

12. Henry Aaron and William B. Schwartz, "Rationing Health Care: The Choice before Us," *Science*, vol. 247 (January 26, 1990), pp. 418–19.

13. See, for example, Stanley B. Jones, "Multiple Choice Health Insurance: The Lessons and Challenge to Private Insurers," *Inquiry*, vol. 27 (Summer 1990), pp. 161–66.

14. Health care spending increased by 11.6 percent between 1989 and 1990 and by 11.1 percent between 1988 and 1989. Gladwell, "Health Costs' Share of GNP Up Sharply"; and Levitt and others, "National Health Care Spending, 1989," p. 118.

15. Northwestern National Life Insurance Company, *Americans Speak Out on Health Care Rationing* (Minneapolis, 1990), p. 18.

16. Daniels, "Why Saying No . . . Is So Hard."

17. David M. Eddy, "What Care is 'Essential'? What Services Are 'Basic'?" *Journal of the American Medical Association*, vol. 265 (February 13, 1991), pp. 782–88.

18. George J. Schieber and Jean-Pierre Poullier, "International Health Spending: Issues and Trends," *Health Affairs*, vol. 10 (Spring 1991), exhibit 3, p. 111.

19. Bengt Jonnson, "What Can Americans Learn from Europeans?" *Health Care Financing Review*, 1989 Annual Supplement, table 8, p. 88.

20. Dale A. Rublee, "Medical Technology in Canada, Germany, and the United States," *Health Affairs*, vol. 8 (Fall 1989), pp. 178–81.

21. Ibid.

22. Frances H. Miller and Graham A. H. Miller, "*The Painful Prescription*: A Procrustean Perspective," *New England Journal of Medicine*, vol. 314 (May 22, 1986), pp. 1383–86.

23. Mark R. Chassin and others, "Does Inappropriate Use Explain Geographic Variations in the Use of Health Care Services?" *Journal of the American Medical Association*, vol. 258 (November 13, 1987), pp. 1–5.

24. Constance M. Winslow and others, "The Appropriateness of Performing Coronary Bypass Surgery," *Journal of the American Medical Association*, vol. 260 (July 22–29, 1988), pp. 505–09. For other studies of inappropriate utilization, see Albert Siu and others, "Inappropriate Use of Hospitals in a Randomized Trial of Health Insurance Plans," *New England Journal of Medicine*, vol. 315 (November 13, 1986), pp. 1259–66; and Robert H. Brook and Mary E. Vaiana, *Appropriateness of Care: A Chart Book* (Washington: National Health Policy Forum, 1989).

25. Rolla Edward Park and others, "Physician Ratings of Appropriate Indi-

cations for Three Procedures: Theoretical Indications vs. Indications Used in Practice," *American Journal of Public Health*, vol. 79 (April 1989), pp. 445–47.

26. Author's calculations using data from George J. Schieber and Jean-Pierre Poullier, "Overview of International Comparisons of Health Care Expenditures," *Health Care Financing Review*, 1989 Annual Supplement, table 4, p. 6.

27. Ibid.

28. Ibid.

29. Daniel Callahan, *Setting Limits: Medical Goals in an Aging Society* (Simon and Schuster, 1987).

30. Anne A. Scitovsky, "Medicare Care in the Last Twelve Months of Life: The Relation between Age, Functional Status, and Medical Expenditures," *Milbank Quarterly*, vol. 66, no. 4 (1988), pp. 640–60.

31. James Lubitz and Ronald Prihoda, "Use and Costs of Medicare Services in the Last Two Years of Life," *Health Care Financing Review*, vol. 5 (Spring 1984), pp. 117–31.

32. Office of Technology Assessment, *Life-Sustaining Technologies and the Elderly* (Washington, 1987), pp. 9, 19.

33. William B. Schwartz and Henry J. Aaron, "A Tough Choice on Health Care Costs," *New York Times*, April 6, 1988, p. A23.

34. Author's calculations based on Daniel R. Waldo and others, "Health Expenditures by Age Group, 1977 and 1987," *Health Care Financing Review*, vol. 10 (Summer 1989), tables 3, 4, pp. 112, 116–18.

35. U.S. Bureau of the Census, *Statistical Abstract of the United States, 1990*, table 13, p. 13.

36. *Cruzan et ux* v. *Director, Missouri Department of Health, et al.*, 497 U.S. 110 (1990).

37. H. Gilbert Welch and Eric B. Larson, "Cost Effectiveness of Bone Marrow Transplantation in Acute Nonlymphocytic Leukemia," *New England Journal of Medicine*, vol. 321 (September 21, 1989), pp. 807–12.

38. Henry J. Aaron and William B. Schwartz, *The Painful Prescription: Rationing Hospital Care* (Brookings, 1984), pp. 29–37.

39. Almost all these strategies can result in health care rationing if stringently enough applied. For example, extremely low hospital reimbursement rates may slow the introduction of certain cost-increasing high technology. Ironically, some cost containment efforts may increase access and reduce rationing. Reducing physician fees, for instance, may lead doctors to increase the number of services provided and the number of patients seen as a way to offset the potential reduction in income.

JEAN I. THORNE

The Oregon Plan Approach to Comprehensive and Rational Health Care

Oregon's Health Plan is one state's proposal for addressing the critical issues relating to health care policy. Many Oregonians have found that, as they talk with people on the national level, there has been a lack of understanding about all the components of their plan. The plan does not focus exclusively on the poor. Rather, it is one that addresses the problems of the 450,000 Oregonians who are currently without health care coverage. It is three interrelated laws that will guarantee health care access for the uninsured in the state. The Oregon Plan clearly outlines the responsibilities of government, employers, employees, and insurers in addressing the needs of the uninsured. Many refer to this proposal as a "rationing" plan, but it does not seem to be so much a rationing plan as a *rational* plan to address the existing health care crisis.

Two years ago, when John Kitzhaber, the president of Oregon's state senate, first presented the concepts of his plan for reform of the health care system in Oregon, no one anticipated the national attention and controversy that would eventually result. Oregon is a small state in the Pacific Northwest—a state that many believe is heavily populated by cowboys and frontiersmen. Its citizens were merely trying to develop a sensible health care financing system for the state. Oregonians had begun to grapple with tough health care issues that many other Americans have apparently preferred not to face—thus, the national attention and the national controversy.

So the Brookings conference was convened to discuss health care rationing. The subtitle of the conference was curious—Opening Pandora's Box? Did it imply that Americans may not want to ration? If so, it is too late. Or did it imply that we may not want to talk about rationing? If so, we are kidding ourselves by pretending that the status quo is an acceptable system.

The stark fact is that more than 32 million Americans have no access to health care. Unless there is cash in hand or contact is made with a benevolent health care provider, those 32 million, in the richest nation on earth, cannot have their pain relieved or their sickness treated. Everyone should realize that Americans have already made decisions to ration health care, but our decisions have been made through a process in which we, as a society, hide and deny ever having made them. The decisions have been made implicitly in a way that merely ignores the faceless and nameless in our society who do not have access to basic care.

Oregon is committed to moving this process from the dark into the light by subjecting it to the noisy debate it deserves. We do not claim that Oregonians have found the perfect cure to the national illness in health care. We do contend that, at the very least, our plan could ease some of the pain and treat some of the sickness now being ignored.

PROBLEMS WITH THE CURRENT SYSTEM

Before describing the plan, I would like to reflect on the current system of health care in this country.

—The percentage of dollars being spent on health care has steadily increased. Today, the United States spends over 12 percent of its GNP on health care—more than any other industrialized nation.

—Although the United States spends more than any other country in the world, its health outcomes do not reflect that standing—witness the U.S. statistics for infant mortality and life expectancy.

—Despite the amount of money spent on health care, there are currently 32 to 37 million Americans who have no health care coverage. These people, especially the poor among them, must fend for themselves, go from doctor to doctor, use money they would normally use for food and shelter, go without care altogether, or wait until they become so seriously ill that they are entitled to receive emergency treatment.

The medicaid program—a program that is supposedly a state-administered federal-state program to cover the health care needs of the poor—has many limitations. Eligibility in the system is not based on need; it is based on category, such as age, family status, or medical condition. Merely being poor and unable to afford medical care is not enough.

—The medicaid system will care for a poor working woman after she becomes pregnant but not before she conceives that child. It ignores her need to be healthy before her child's conception. It further ignores her need to remain healthy after her child is born.

—The system offers total coverage for a poor five-year-old, but not necessarily to that child's eight-year-old sister or brother. It denies even the most basic services to a poor child who was not born after some magical date established in federal law (September 30, 1983).

—The system statutorily excludes poor men and women without children from coverage, regardless of how impoverished and destitute they may be.

—The system tells a poor woman that she can no longer have her health care needs covered under medicaid because her youngest child is now out of school. This means that her child is no longer dependent, and that she is therefore no longer in a "family with dependent children."

—The system requires that everything—even treatments of questionable efficacy—be given to those who fit into the proper category, while it completely ignores even the most basic health care needs of those poor who are not of the correct age, sex, or family composition.

Certainly none of this constitutes "health care rationing," does it?

The federal Office of Management and Budget recently announced that it was undertaking a "crash study" to determine the reason that medicaid expenditures have gone through the roof over the past few years. Across the nation, states are struggling with this astronomical growth. What are some of the methods states are using to contain these costs? The options are limited—cut people from the program, eliminate entire categories of services, place limits on the number of physician visits or pharmacy dispensings, or cut provider reimbursement. All these are legal; all are arbitrary, but it certainly is not rationing, is it?

The current system can allow us to spend incredible amounts of money. The sky, not our pocketbooks, is the limit as far as medical possibilities are concerned. By spending increasing amounts of money on health care with no corresponding increase in health, we are forced to take funds away from other services that can have as much, if not more, of an impact on the health of our citizens—services such as housing, public safety, and education.

Everyone is certainly aware of the questionable benefits of certain procedures; yet, those involved in medicaid can do little to control their use. The ability to deny a service is limited, because a patient can almost always find a doctor who will say that a certain procedure is medically necessary, or that it may be of value.

OREGON'S PLAN

In Oregon, discussions were conducted about the current problems with its health care system, and it was decided that there had to be a better way. The initial public discussions about trade-offs in health policy began during Oregon's 1987 legislative session. Oregon lawmakers decided that, given the high cost and low success rate for various organ transplants in the medicaid program, and the number of poor Oregonians with no access to health care coverage, the state would be better off spending its available dollars differently. Although the legislature entitled more poor Oregonians to coverage under the medicaid program, it eliminated transplant coverage for those already eligible for medicaid.

The impact of that decision was not truly felt until months later, when a young boy died who might have benefited from a bone marrow transplant. The boy was on medicaid. The death of Coby Howard forced Oregonians to openly face the conflict between unlimited possibilities in health care and limited resources. Massive media attention to his death forced an emotional, difficult debate. During the next year, various legislative committees, advocacy groups, and citizens concerned with the issues in health care made known the inequities and problems in the current system. The result was the Oregon Health Plan.

The plan advanced and passed by the 1989 legislature is one that was developed and supported by a wide-ranging coalition of labor, business, consumers, and providers. It is not a plan of either right-wing extremists or left-wing radicals; it has bipartisan support. It is a plan that states as a matter of public policy a person's right to health care, but one that also recognizes that there are limits to what society can publicly support. It requires painful and explicit choices. It is a plan that will allow government to buy more health for the health care dollar.

Before describing the portion of the Oregon Plan relating to medicaid—apparently the most controversial part—I touch briefly on the other two laws passed by the Oregon legislature. These are the pieces of the plan that seem to be unknown but that will affect even more Oregonians than the part relating to medicaid.

One piece of Oregon's program already in place is a high-risk pool for the medically uninsurable. These are the people with severe health care needs who cannot buy the coverage to take care of those needs; they must go without care or have much of it subsidized through a cost shift. This part of the plan is now funded through a combination of insurance assessments and participant premiums. Although available funding currently limits the program to one thousand participants, its size is projected to double within the next two years.

The second, and perhaps most important, part of the plan relates to employer responsibilities. The law requires that by 1995 all employers in Oregon must provide health care coverage to their employees and dependents. The benefit package to be covered must, at a minimum, be comparable to that which the medicaid population will receive. Although normally not supportive of increased mandates on employers, medium and large businesses were strongly supportive of this part of the plan. They supported it because they saw that they were already footing the bill through cost-shifting of those who were uninsured.

Finally, the centerpiece of Oregon's plan is the law that would revamp the state's medicaid program. The elements of the plan are quite simple. It would cover all persons under 100 percent of the federal poverty level, regardless of their age, medical condition, or family structure; guarantee them a benefit package that will focus on those services with the greatest impact on their health; deliver those benefits through managed care—a system that will ensure access, quality care, and cost containment; and pay for those services at reasonable rates, which would reduce or eliminate the cost shift.

It is the second element—the design of the benefit package—that seems to have stirred the national interest. There has long been talk in America about basic benefits, but there has been no determination of a common definition of what that constitutes.

Oregon confronts the current reality of health care in America with an explicit, rational, public process for defining an affordable, quality package of health care benefits. The process is governed by the Health Services Commission, an eleven-member panel composed of physicians, consumers, and other medical professionals appointed by

the governor. The commission has had the formidable task of prioritizing health care services "based on the comparable benefits to the
population to be served."

This massive undertaking has never before been tried. Under the
glare of a national spotlight, the commissioners worked through their
historic task. It has been a difficult process, for although no one ever
welcomes a public stumble, this process was specifically and inten-
tionally designed to be open.

It might be helpful to have a brief overview of the prioritization
process used by the commission. The commission received public input from forty-seven community meetings, twelve public hearings,
and a thousand-person telephone survey regarding the values Oregonians believe should guide public policy decisions on health care.
Commissioners used this input, as well as their own judgment, to
develop and rank seventeen categories of care (see table 1 in Michael
Garland's paper). For example, the top priority category is for acute
fatal conditions, where treatment allows full recovery. Other examples of the seventeen categories include preventive care for children, preventive care for adults, and maternity care. Also included is
a category for services in which treatment causes minimal or no improvement in the quality of life.

The commission defined 709 condition-treatment pairs and assigned them to the various categories. The condition-treatment pairs
were then ranked within the categories according to their net benefit—that is, the degree to which a person's well-being would improve
by receiving that treatment for that given condition. Finally, the commission used its judgment to move specific condition-treatment pairs
up or down the list, according to their costs and public value.

The work of the commission was an example of citizen involvement
in government at its best. These volunteers spent eighteen months of
their lives, at least twenty hours per week per commissioner, devoted
to compiling a list that made sense. Many other Oregonians gave their
time, by providing expert testimony or by organizing community
meetings. It is estimated that altogether more than twenty-five thousand volunteer hours were spent on the final product.

The commission did an extremely creditable job. Those who have
reviewed the list have found little to criticize. This list, along with an
actuarial report that prices it at various levels, was delivered to the
governor and legislature in May 1991. Lawmakers cannot alter the

list. They can and must determine where to draw the line on which listed services will constitute the standard benefit package.

The Health Services Commission, through its deliberations, presented recommendations to assist lawmakers in making the tough decisions about where to draw the line. The commission recommended that for the most part the services in the first nine categories be regarded as "essential" to a basic health plan and be funded. The next four categories considered "very important," were to be funded to the greatest extent possible. The last four categories, though acknowledged to be valuable to certain individuals, were felt to be of less importance to society as a whole or of questionable benefit.

Those services above the line drawn by the legislature will be covered for the current and expanded group of eligible clients; those services below the line will not. The legislature responded to the recommendations of the commission and appropriated funds to cover the top 587 items on the 709-item list. This means that diagnostic services, preventive and primary care, and other effective treatments will be covered. Those types of treatments not covered are mostly ones that are not as effective or may, in fact, be futile.

If revenues fall short, lawmakers cannot, as they usually do, arbitrarily cut people from the program or arbitrarily cut what is paid to medical providers. Their only options are to raise more money or to reduce the service level. This will require explicit decisions about *what* is covered, not implicit and hidden decisions that affect *who* is covered.

There will never be an opportunity to implement this program unless substantial waivers of federal medicaid law are received. Once work was completed on the benefit package by legislatively drawing the line, a waiver request was submitted (August 1991). A demonstration project is possible with the permission of the secretary of Health and Human Services. Considering that it will take six months to introduce the program after the necessary waivers are granted, implementation is currently planned for July 1992.

CRITICISMS AND OREGON'S RESPONSES

Many criticisms of Oregon's plan have surfaced at the national level. The following are the principal ones.

1. *Medical procedures cannot be prioritized. A formula cannot adequately*

consider the importance of medicine. I address the second part of that criticism first. In 1990 the commission produced its first work product—one that was labeled by many as the "first list" and later called "the first list that was quickly dumped." The commissioners had explored using a strict cost-benefit ratio, but the first computer run revealed the shortcomings of that approach.

Commissioners found that the formula could not take into account the values of Oregonians or allow them to use their own judgments regarding what might be either important or reasonable. The commission took the time to revise its methodology so that values and judgment were primary components of the process. Ultimately, the commissioners did produce what appears to be a reasonable list.

2. *This list means that people whose condition falls near the bottom will go without care*. It is important to remember that a given diagnosis may have several treatments on the list. Let me use HIV disease as an example. High on the list are treatment for the early stages of HIV and treatment for opportunistic infections. Also high on the list is a very important category the commission labeled "comfort care." Comfort care allows for pain management and home-based services for those in the end stages of a terminal disease, such as cancer or AIDS. But very low, almost at the end of the list, is aggressive treatment of the end stages of HIV. What the ranking on the list reflects is the values of Oregonians: compassionate care is often better than aggressive treatment that offers little or no hope for improvement in the quality of life.

3. *Oregon only needs to spend more money*. There are plans to spend more money for medical care in medicaid under this program. But rather than do it in wasteful ways that are perfectly legal under current law but that have little chance of improving the health of the poor, Oregonians wish to do it sensibly. Instead of merely paying more and covering everything for the select group of poor who fit within the "right category," Oregonians wish to assure all poor people that they will be guaranteed coverage for a package of care that should make a difference in their lives.

4. *Oregon is rationing care to the poor*. First of all, it is important to note that what is currently being done throughout the nation is rationing poor people, not services to the poor. The United States denies virtually all care to many of the poor, while righteously providing a full package of benefits to some of the poor.

Then, it must be remembered that the standard benefit package developed through this process will also become the required basic package for those covered under the employer mandates. Many of the services high on the list may be those not currently covered under many employer-based plans, such as preventive care to children and adults and preventive dental services.

5. *Oregon is rationing care to poor women and children.* This argument seems to ignore the fact that the majority of the poor Oregonians who will gain access to health care through the expanded medicaid program are poor women and children. These are the poor women and children who currently receive no coverage because they do not qualify for medicaid under any of the proper categories—the woman whose child is no longer "dependent," the son whose birth date falls before the "magic date" in federal law, and the single woman with a chronic illness who is not yet pregnant. These are the poor women and children who will be guaranteed coverage under our program.

The prioritized health services list itself also stresses providing important and effective health services to women and children. High on the list are checkups, immunizations, maternity care, care for the newborn, and treatment for virtually all childhood diseases. Oregon will be covering all mandated and optional service categories under medicaid law. But rather than provide reimbursement for every potential treatment under these service categories because a practitioner argues that someone "might potentially" benefit, Oregon is tying its coverage policy to treatments that are known to be truly effective.

Not only will these services be guaranteed to those women and children who are poor, but they will also serve as the basis for the standard benefit package available through the employer mandates. This ensures health care coverage to the growing number of working low-income women and their children who do not qualify for medicaid.

Perhaps the biggest frustration in trying to move forward with the Oregon proposal is dealing with critics who seem only to ask, "How is Oregon's plan less than perfect?" It is these critics who examine isolated components of the plan without looking more broadly at how they fit within an overall policy objective. Are those who oppose the plan contending that the current "system" of health care financing is perfect? Do they contend that the current system is rational, equitable, or affordable?

Would it not seem fairer to examine the ways in which the Oregon Plan is better than what is currently in place than to hold it up to some unattainable ideal for which no one has yet developed a plan?

Frequently, the resistance to the Oregon Plan, especially in Washington, D.C., seems to be not so much a resistance to the plan as a resistance to having to make a decision. Many would prefer to see Oregon and its plan dry up and go away than to be forced to confront the current system and the political forces behind that system. Many have fought hard for the federal mandates and do not believe a state should be allowed to question them. They resist changes that might threaten those successes or change the status quo.

Oregonians are finding themselves caught in a catch-22. On the one hand, there are those lawmakers who say that we had better pump substantial amounts of new money into our program so that few, if any, services for the current medicaid population would be eliminated. On the other hand, there are those lawmakers and officials who contend that our program must be budget neutral, not requiring any more federal dollars than might be spent under the current system. And there are probably many who would hope that we would become so caught up in these conflicting goals that no tough policy decisions will have to be made.

CONCLUSION

In Oregon, those tough decisions have been and will be made. The answers to the health care crisis are not simple. They are not without controversy and they are not without emotion. Americans must understand that the only escape from controversy and emotion on this issue is a fantasy world in which they pretend that there are not really 32 million Americans without access to basic health care.

Oregonians believe we have an answer. We do not pretend that it is perfect. But while others wait for someone else to come up with the perfect solution, they continue to deny the existence of those 32 million Americans. The status quo is not an answer. In Oregon, we are tired of waiting for others to develop the solution to our health care problems. We do not see a national answer on the horizon.

Until there is agreement on a national plan, states should be given an opportunity to try different approaches. And that is what Oregonians ask. We want the opportunity to make our plan work. Through it, we believe we can dig into Pandora's box and provide hope—hope to those Oregonians who currently must go without access to basic care.

Policy Questions

MICHAEL J. GARLAND

Rationing in Public: Oregon's Priority-Setting Methodology

The Oregon Basic Health Services Act,* with its priority-setting cen-terpiece, is an example of what Daniel Bell calls nonmarket decision-making.[1] These are collective choices that simply cannot be success-fully pursued by multiple individuals making rational purchases in the marketplace. These choices must result from political processes. They must involve other members of the community besides individ-ual buyers and sellers in determining the value of specific goods or services. Health care programs that rely on third-party financing, es-pecially those aimed at serving the nation's poor, require just that kind of decisionmaking. The choices at stake involve not only the poor but the whole community, because they ultimately concern guarantees from all of us to all of us about the quality of our life in common. The need for choice challenges everyone to envision and enact a fairer, more functional, more prudent, more compassionate, more effective, and more efficient health care system.

The Oregon approach is based on three central ethical commit-ments that the methodology seeks to serve: first, that it is more equi-table to assure everyone basic health care than to offer a larger, but unevaluated, collection of benefits to some of the poor while exclud-ing others from anything but emergency care; second, that explicit, publicly accountable choice is better than the hidden rationing that now occurs; third, that health care priorities should combine authen-tic community values with expert technical judgments about health

*Three statutes passed in 1989 constitute the Oregon Basic Health Services Act: SB 27 reforms medicaid and creates the Health Services Commission; SB 935 creates incentives for small businesses to make health insurance available to employees; SB 534 provides funding for a high-risk pool to make insurance available at near-market prices for persons otherwise unable to obtain insur-ance in the open market.

services. At the heart of the Oregon approach is a prioritized list of health services that is to be used by the Oregon legislature to guide medicaid budget decisions. The list is also supposed to guide benefit package choices for private insurance plans that are to be made available to small businesses and to persons currently uninsurable in the private insurance market. The methodology for public decisionmaking that is built into the Oregon statutes and further elaborated by the Health Services Commission merits careful, critical examination by other states struggling with the same need for nonmarket decisionmaking.

My discussion of the priority-setting methodology focuses on the content of the priorities list, the basic four-step process within which the list functions, the specific priority-setting process developed by the Oregon Health Services Commission, and the most common criticisms of the Oregon strategy.[2]

THE LIST

Before the list was produced by the Health Services Commission, the debate about the Oregon Plan was totally theoretical and highly, if not wildly, conjectural. Some early critics asserted that the task of setting health services priorities is too complex, and that only nonsense could be produced in the short time frame and with the methods proposed.[3] A list exists now, and it should be inspected and criticized for what it is, not for what theoretical arguments predicted it would be.

Other early critics declared a priori that the method was vitiated by injustice.[4] The reasoning was that because the laws established a program that rationed health care exclusively for the poor, any list could only be an instrument of injustice, and therefore the process should be immediately aborted. In fact, the list was intended to be an aid for making decisions, not only about budgets and state tax dollars but also about the meaning of community and fairness in Oregon. In the legislation that initiated the process, the state made a new commitment to the poor, both those served by medicaid and those who would benefit from increased access to private health insurance at their places of employment. That the process was immediately called theoretically unjust because it was directed at the poor is best answered by observing what the legislature did with the list. Contrary to predictions, the legislature's actual use of the list brought significant new dollars into the medicaid budget, enlarging the state's commitment to secure adequate access to health care for the poor.

The Structure of the List

The entire list comprises 709 items, each of which consists of a health condition paired with one or more treatments likely to be used in providing care to a patient with that condition or diagnosis. The commissioners created a system of seventeen categories to organize the items logically, placed the categories into priority order, and then rank-ordered the items within each category. The categories are fashioned around values that the commission elicited from the public through forty-seven community meetings and twelve public hearings. The categories constitute the basic zones of priority on the list, with category 1 being the highest-priority group of services. The categories may also be viewed as being *disease-oriented* or *health-oriented*, as indicated in table 1. The categories overlap somewhat because certain items that conceptually belong in a given category have special characteristics that led the commissioners to place them above or below their "logical" position.

In transmitting the list to the legislature, the commissioners identified three large sections of the list as having different importance for collectively funded health care and made some recommendations.[5] Categories 1 to 9 must be funded because they are essential components of basic health care; categories 10 to 13 should be funded to the greatest extent possible because they are considered very important elements of health care; and categories 14 to 17 should be funded as resources permit because they are valuable to individuals, but significantly less likely to be cost-effective or to produce substantial benefits.

The 1991 legislature passed a budget for medicaid that funds the program through line 587, which includes virtually all (98 percent) of the services in the "essential to basic care" section, most (82 percent) of the services in the "very important" section, and a few (7 percent) of the services in the "valuable to individuals but of minimal gain and/or high cost" section.[6] The items that logically belonged to the essential-to-basic-care group of categories but remain unfunded (9 of 366

TABLE 1. *Health Services Commission Priorities by Categories*

Disease oriented	Rank	Health oriented
Fatal conditions		
Treatment prevents death with		
Full recovery 1		
	2.	Maternity and newborn care
Residual problems 3		
	4.	Preventive care for children
Treatment extends life and		
improves quality of life 5		
	6.	Reproductive services
Treatment gives comfort care. 7		
	8.	Preventive dental care
	9.	Adult preventive care (I)
Nonfatal conditions		
Acute condition		
Treatment provides		
full cure 10		
Chronic condition		
Single treatment		
improves quality of life 11		
Acute condition		
Treatment achieves partial		
recovery 12		
Chronic condition		
Repeated treatments improve		
quality of life 13		
Acute, self limiting condition		
Treatment speeds recovery 14		
	15.	Infertility treatments
	16.	Adult preventive care (II)
Fatal or nonfatal conditions		
Treatments provide minimal or		
no improvement in length or		
quality of life 17		

Source: Adapted from Oregon Health Services Commission, *Prioritization of Health Services*, appendix G, pp. 11–12.

condition-treatment pairs) are ones that the commissioners judged would have a very poor potential for success.

Examples of Categories[7]

1. Acute, fatal conditions for which treatment prevents death and provides full recovery—for example, repair of deep open wound of the neck; appendectomy; medical therapy for myocarditis.

2. Maternity care, including disorders of the newborn—for example, obstetrical care; medical therapy for drug reactions and intoxications specific to newborns; medical therapy for low birth weight babies.

3. Acute, fatal conditions for which treatment prevents death but recovery is limited—for example, surgical treatment for head injury with prolonged loss of consciousness; medical therapy for acute bacterial meningitis; reduction of an open fracture of a joint.

4. Prevention care for children—for example, immunizations; medical therapy for streptococcal sore throat and scarlet fever; screening for specific problems such as vision or hearing problems or anemia.

5. Chronic conditions that are fatal and for which treatment improves life span and the quality of life—for example, medical therapy for type I Diabetes Mellitus; medical and surgical treatment for treatable cancer of the uterus; medical therapy for asthma.

6. Reproductive services—for example, contraceptive management, vasectomy; tubal ligation.

7. Comfort care—for example, palliative therapy for conditions in which death is imminent.

8. Preventive dental care for adults and children—for example, cleaning; fluoride treatments.

9. Preventive care for adults (I)—for example, mammograms; blood pressure screening; medical therapy and chemoprophylaxis for primary tuberculosis.

10. Acute, nonfatal conditions for which treatment is likely to bring a return to previous health—for example, medical therapy for acute thyroiditis; medical therapy for vaginitis; restorative dental service for caries.

11. Chronic, nonfatal conditions for which a one-time treatment improves the quality of life—for example, hip replacement; laser surgery for diabetic retinopathy; medical therapy for rheumatic fever.

12. Acute, nonfatal conditions for which treatment is unable to fully restore previous health—for example, arthroscopic repair of internal derangement of knee; repair of corneal laceration.

13. Chronic, nonfatal conditions for which repetitive treatment improves the quality of life—for example, medical therapy for chronic sinusitis, migraine headaches, psoriasis.

14. Acute conditions that are nonfatal and self-limited, for which treatment expedites recovery—for example, medical therapy for diaper rash, acute conjunctivitis, pharyngitis.

15. Infertility services—for example, medical therapy for anovulation; microsurgery for tubal disease; in-vitro fertilization.

16. Preventive services for adults (II)—for example, dipstick urinalysis for hematuria in adults under 60 years of age; sigmoidoscopy for persons under 40 years of age; screening of nonpregnant adults for Type I Diabetes Mellitus.

17. Fatal or nonfatal conditions for which treatment provides minimal or no improvement in quality of life—for example, repair fingertip avulsion that does not include fingernail; medical therapy for gallstones without cholecystitis; medical therapy for viral warts.

THE FOUR-STEP PROCESS

An essential, and often overlooked, feature of the general methodology of the Basic Health Services Act is its segmentation into four distinct steps, with a division of tasks and responsibilities among the commission, the legislature, and specific agencies (see figure 1). In the first step of the process, the Health Services Commission was required to develop a list of health service priorities based on community values about health care and on technical information about the effectiveness of various health services relative to the needs of the population to be served. Step one was completed in May 1991, when the commission delivered the list, together with actuarial estimates of the cost of funding different priority levels, to the governor and the legislature. That triggered step two, at which the full legislature, using the list as a decision guide, had the task of setting budgets that established de facto the benefit package to be offered by the new Oregon Medicaid Program. This package will also become the norm that must be substantially contained in any private health insurance plan offered under the aegis of the small business and high-risk insurance

FIGURE 1. *Oregon's Priority-Setting Process*

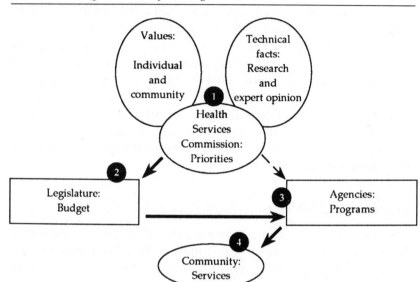

programs. Step two was completed during the 1991 session of the legislature, which finished its budget allocations and adjourned at the end of June.

The third step in the process provides the relevant agencies (medicaid, Oregon Medical Insurance Pool Board, and High Risk Insurance Pool Governing Board) with the budget decision that creates the benefit package for medicaid and associated private insurance packages. The first essential administrative task was for the Office of Medical Assistance Programs to request necessary waivers of several federal medicaid regulations. Without approval from the Health Care Financing Administration (HCFA), the medicaid portion of the plan cannot be implemented. The waiver request went to the HCFA in August 1991, with a response expected by the spring of 1992.

At step three the agencies must also put in place all the administrative and evaluation elements necessary to run a complex social program. Figure 1 shows a secondary arrow from the Health Services Commmission (HSC) to the agencies because part of the concept of the process is for the agencies to use the priority list to guide administrative decisions so that the new programs will be a consistent expression of the values on which the priorities are based.

The fourth step is the actual implementation of new service programs in the community. These services involve all persons at or below 100 percent of the federal poverty level (that is, by the 1991 standard, an income of $928 per month for a family of three) who will be declared eligible for medicaid. Those with incomes above 100 percent of the federal poverty level (unless already included in a mandated categorical program for medicaid) will be served through either of the two health insurance pools. At this step, the ultimate goals of improved access to adequate health care depend on the ability of agencies to maintain cooperative relations with direct care providers. If the HCFA grants the necessary waivers, Oregon will begin phasing in the new medicaid program in July 1992.

Prioritization Methodology: Values—Individual and Community

In any rational decisionmaking process, whether it is an individual choice like selecting a new car or a public choice like funding health care for the poor, prioritization consists of combining values with technical facts (or, in the absence of facts, expert opinion). Using public hearings, structured community meetings, and a telephone survey, the HSC solicited two kinds of value data: *individual* values and *community* values. The primary source of the individual value data was a random-sample telephone survey of the Oregon population using an instrument adapted from Kaplan's quality-of-well-being scale (QWB).[8] (The QWB scale is discussed in Robert Kaplan's paper.) The function of the solicitation of individual value statements is to provide a scale for weighting the outcomes of health care in terms of benefit to patients, described as quality-of-life factors.

These aggregated values are two steps removed from the individualistic focus of informed consent in clinical encounters. Respondents were not immediately experiencing symptoms but were asked to project their feelings hypothetically. Individual responses were then aggregated so that a mean number was taken to stand for all the individual valuations of different levels of quality of life. Thus, the QWB weights do not represent actual patients' expressions of value about conditions but do give projected estimates. The aggregation of these estimates fits the task of resource planning, which must make available those services most likely to serve the community's most important quality-of-life goals when people seek assistance from the health care system.

Community values were solicited for the HSC by special arrangement with Oregon Health Decisions (OHD), a nonprofit organization that has existed since 1983 to facilitate public involvement in the development of health policy about ethical issues confronting society. The goal of the community meetings was to generate for the HSC publicly examined statements about what makes health care "important to us" as a common good. Participants were asked to think and express themselves in the first person plural—that is, as members of a statewide community for whom health care has a shared value.

Forty-seven community meetings were held throughout the state—all counties but two—from January through March 1990. A total of 1,048 citizens participated. Each meeting aimed at discovering the local consensus about community values regarding health care. The method for these meetings produced a separation of facts and values through structured small group discussions that called for individual judgments about priorities among a list of nine categories of health services, discussion among participants to identify values underlying their priority judgments, and identification by the group of key shared values about health care. The next step was to identify principal values from each of the small groups to determine which value themes would constitute an "authentic message" to the HSC from the particular geographic community. Reports from these community meetings were collated and summarized by OHD staff into the final report for the HSC.[9]

The meetings identified a constellation of thirteen value themes about health care. These themes represent the multidimensional quality of community values about health care. The value themes were not prioritized either by the communities or by the OHD staff. Without implying any priority order or weight, the themes displayed in table 2 summarize the "message from the communities" to the HSC. The table gives a short label for each value theme followed by a brief elaboration of the meanings typically included in community discussions.

The community values were instrumental in bringing several important themes into the HSC deliberation. The establishment of seventeen categories as the primary determinant of priority within the list is directly linked to the commission's response to the values expressed in the community meetings and to the testimony provided at the twelve public hearings presided over by the commissioners. The

TABLE 2. *Value Themes from Community Meetings*

Label	Value significance for community
Prevention	Avoiding harm and suffering, improving quality of life, exercising wisdom and personal choice
Quality of life	Attending to emotional well-being, pain and suffering, independence, functional capacity
Cost-effectiveness	Seeking wise investments in health
Ability to function	Restoring emotional well-being, productivity, independence, and general quality of life
Equity	Contributing to the fairness of community life
Effectiveness of treatment	Preferring to fund treatments known to work
Benefits many	Seeking to treat problems that affect a large proportion of the community
Mental health and chemical dependency	Connecting mental and physical health, supporting functional ability and productivity
Personal choice	Preserving autonomy and personal dignity
Community compassion	Seeking to ensure humane response to the terminally ill and other vulnerable persons
Impact on society	Attending to effects on others from treating (or not treating) certain health problems
Length of life	Acknowledging that life is necessary to realize any values
Personal responsibility	Encouraging individual autonomy and control over one's own health status

structure of the list in the final report of the commission clearly exhibits a major impact attributable to these "soundings" of community values.

Prioritization Methodology: Ranking of Categories

The use of a ranked set of categories is the HSC's primary mechanism for deciding priorities among health services.[10] After the categories were created and rank-ordered, a net benefit formula was used to establish priority order among individual condition-treatment pairs within each category. The ranking process consisted of five steps.

First, a list of categories was created that was judged capable of containing all condition-treatment pairs. The list drew on ideas derived from the community meetings and public hearings, from commissioners' intuitive habits of thought, and from the literature on health care.[11]

Second, the community value themes were arranged into three broad value attributes: *value to society*—defined as comprising the values of prevention, benefit to many, impact on society, quality-of-life impact, personal responsibility, cost-effectiveness, community compassion, and response to mental health and chemical dependency problems; *value to an individual at risk of needing the service*—defined as comprising the values of prevention, quality of life, ability to function, length of life, personal responsibility, equity, effectiveness of treatment, personal choice, community compassion, and response to mental health and chemical dependency problems; and *essential to a basic health care package*—defined as comprising the values of prevention, benefit to many, quality-of-life impact, cost-effectiveness, and impact on society.

Third, the attributes were given a "perspective weight" unique to each commissioner. Each commissioner distributed 100 points among the three attributes. Thus, commissioner A might have given value to society 40 points, value to the individual 20 points, and essential to basic health care 40 points. Next, the commissioners, using a 1 to 10 scale, individually scored each service category in terms of the three attributes. Thus, commissioner A in considering the category of maternity care might have scored it 9 for value to society, 8 for value to the individual, and 10 for essential to basic health care.

Fourth, after individually scoring each category, the commissioners engaged in an open discussion session (modified Delphi technique) to examine the reasons for differences among their scores in the various categories. In this discussion, it was particularly apparent that the commissioners felt obliged to make their judgments as "instructed representatives" of the community, referring repeatedly to the community meetings and public hearings to interpret their scores to one another.[12] After the commissioners were afforded the opportunity to alter their scores, the final scores were multiplied by the appropriate perspective weights, and the mean weighted score for each category was determined.

Fifth, the rank order among the categories was based on the mean score for each category (the sum of the weighted scores divided by the number of commissioners).

Some critics of the Oregon process have questioned whether the community meetings and public hearings actually had any effect on the prioritization process.[13] The point of the criticism is to cast doubt on the claim that this process has an authentic connection to the values expressed at the community meetings and public hearings. Although the connection between the community values and the priorities list is not easily traceable, the process of category ranking is where the connection is located. There can be no doubt that the commissioners thought they were responding to the values garnered from their consultations with the public. They structured their category-ranking process to make these values central to the priorities, and they repeatedly referred to the community meetings data in their consensus discussions that were a critical part of the process. There is no evidence to support the suspicion that the community meetings and public hearings had no effect on the commission's work. The evidence, in fact, indicates just the opposite.[14]

Prioritization Methodology: Technical Facts and Expert Opinion

From fifty-four panels of health care providers, the HSC solicited outcome-of-treatment information. Because treatment occurs in response to a condition, the information was solicited in terms of condition-treatment pairs developed from ICD–9 (*International Classification of Disease*) or DSM-III-R (*Diagnostic and Statistical Manual of Mental Disorders*) codes and related to CPT–4 (*Current Physician's Terminology*) or ADA (American Dental Association) codes for treatments. Providers were requested to provide: (1) median age at onset of diagnosis; (2) probability that the designated treatment would be used; (3) expected duration of benefits from the treatment; (4) outcome probabilities with and without treatment; and (5) cost to payer with and without treatment. Outcomes were to be identified in five columns: (1) death; (2–4) residual effects; and (5) asymptomatic cure. Each column asked for a probability estimate of the occurrence of a particular outcome. The "residual effects" columns were to have a probability figure designating the major symptom or impairment of physical or social activity or personal mobility (QWB factors). Providers responded in terms of a reference list of twenty-four symptoms and six measures of activity (two each for mobility, physical activity, and social activity).

Prioritization Methodology: Net-Benefit Formula

The commission used the individual value weights (QWB) and the outcomes data from providers in a net-benefit formula that initially was expected to be the primary instrument for prioritization. Eventually, however, the formula became a secondary element, being used to establish an ordering within the categories that had been previously placed in priority order using the category-ranking methodology just described. Initially, the formula produced a cost-benefit ratio. In the final application, however, only a net-benefit ratio was used, with consideration given to cost information when commissioners questioned an item's position on the list or when the net-benefit formula produced a tie between items.[15]

The net-benefit ratio is obtained by subtracting the probable outcome if a condition was not treated from the probable outcome of treating a given condition. All outcomes were expressed in terms of QWB factors. The expert panels provided the probability estimates.

It should be noted that cost of treatment data proved to be so difficult to acquire reliably that their use was abandoned except to break ties when net-benefit scores were identical within the same category. A persistent misunderstanding of the prioritization process is the belief that a cost-benefit or cost-effectiveness ratio was the primary determinant of position on the list. But, as mentioned, reliable data proved so difficult to acquire that ultimately costs were used only to make marginal adjustments in a small number of the items on the list.

The net-benefit formula was used to rank-order items within each category. After this was accomplished, the commissioners went through the entire list line by line to identify any items that intuitively seemed "out of place." Commissioners who wanted to move an item on the list were held to a "reasonableness" test, which consisted of evaluating the public health impact, the cost of medical treatment, the incidence of the condition, the effectiveness of treatment, social costs, and cost of nontreatment to justify a different position on the list. These justifications were made in open discussion, with the final determination resting on consensus. The commissioners also sought to follow a rule of placing services with a preventive effect ahead of items referring to the same diagnosis in a severe or exacerbated stage.

The list, together with actuarial estimates of the aggregate costs of funding benefit packages at various levels of depth in the list, was used by the Oregon legislature to guide budgetary decisions during the 1991 session. The legislature, as has been noted, surprised many critics by voting substantial new dollars to the medicaid expansion program and funding the list through line 587.

PRIORITIES AND ETHICAL CONCERNS

The central premise of the Oregon Plan is the idea that by using a prioritized list of health services to guide legislative budget decisions and administrative actions, an ethically acceptable basic benefit package could be defined that would securely include those services considered most important, and focus marginal decisions on services of lesser importance. The moral goal of setting priorities is to rationally carry out the state's commitment to securing access to health care for the poor.

Five themes of ethical concern have been raised by observers of the evolving Oregon Plan both inside and outside the state. First, because of its primary focus on medicaid recipients and the currently uninsured population, and because the legislative package made no front-end commitment of new dollars to pay for expanded access, the plan had been labeled unfair to the poor,[16] and particularly to women and children who are major recipients of medicaid support.[17] This concern is heightened by the fact that the staging of the Oregon Plan initially exempts from prioritization those medicaid services now offered to the elderly, the blind, and the disabled. At the heart of this criticism is the view that if allocation or explicit rationing of health services is ever to be considered ethical, it must include everyone, rich and poor alike. It is fundamentally unfair, these critics say, to expand access for poor persons by rationing care only among the poorest members of society, which is, in effect, asking only the poor to bear the burden of expanding access.[18]

This concern highlights a fundamental challenge faced by Oregon as a civic community—that is, how to achieve greater *equity* in the distribution of benefits and, at the same time, *fairly* distribute the burden of producing improved equity. Undoubtedly, the most frequent—and most passionate—objections to the plan are made in the name of justice and fairness. These criticisms have a common theoretical ideal: rationing that involves everyone is more equitable than rationing aimed only at the poor.

The problem with insisting on a theoretical ideal is that the government does not have the level of control over the entire range of third-party systems needed to implement the imagined universal rationing program. State government, however, now does have control over, and responsibility for, programs aimed at providing access to health care for the poor. Rationalizing that part of the system in pursuit of greater equity is an appropriate goal of state health policy. Policy developments at this level need to be judged in terms of current political dynamics and their capacity to contribute to more ideal long-term solutions.

Leonard Fleck, in a constructive analysis, argues that the Oregon focus on medicaid and private insurance for low-income workers is fair even to current medicaid-eligible persons, even though a more ideal rationing scheme would include all income levels. This argument for fairness rests on the proposition that persons now eligible for medicaid would be making a rational choice to forgo some lesser benefits to gain greater assurance that they would have access to private health insurance in a low-paying job—a situation they are likely to face as they move from medicaid eligibility to greater financial independence.[19] This hypothetical rationality is proposed as the basis for considering the Oregon Plan just—albeit nonideal.

Fleck acknowledges what many other justice-centered criticisms overlook. They fault the Oregon Plan, not because it involves *rationing*, but because the rationing occurs in circumstances that are *not ideal*. This provides for clear and forceful theoretical argumentation, but in the end only dimly illuminates policy decisions that must be made in present, less-than-ideal circumstances. Medicaid budgets, for example, have to be dealt with in both the long term and the short term. The plight of persons without health insurance who need health care requires prompt response. The only way to ration to everyone at the same time is to have already put in place a system of universal guarantees and to have governmental control over all parts of the system. This kind of ideal thinking leaps over the problem that governments and the uninsured face right now.

The real value for public policy from arguments based on ideal justice is their capacity to keep us all uncomfortable with solutions that, though they may be improvements over current injustice, remain less just than other conceivable solutions. Daniels, in his critique, acknowledges this tension and concludes that it is a matter of "political judgment" whether the pursuit of a "lesser justice" is likely to lead to further reforms (and closer to ideal justice) or, conversely, to hinder the quest for greater equity.[20] Although Daniels makes a distinction between *ethical* and *political* judgment, it must be noted that the latter in the daily life of any civic community is the only available engine of ethical *action*. If ethical judgments are to have public effect, they must be linked with political judgment.

A second concern raised by critical observers is that the plan may seriously corrupt community spirit by legitimizing a mean-spirited attitude toward the poor.[21] This criticism sees priority-based allocations as ethically proper only if everyone in the community is at risk of having to live with the results of a priority system to be used to allocate resources. It is considered destructive of the moral basis of society to legitimize restrictions on health care for the poor while permitting the more affluent to indulge in extravagant life-styles, including excessive use of health services that are financed by collective resources such as private health insurance.

This concern is often attached to criticisms of the community meetings that were organized by Oregon Health Decisions to generate a report on community values to be used by the HSC in setting priorities. Daniels is suspicious of the results of the meetings because only health services for the poor, and not those for the majority, would be affected by the values expressed at the meetings and reported to the HSC.[22] He believes this bias was compounded later, when the legislature, using the priorities based on these values, implemented its task of setting a budget—again affecting health care for the poor, but not for the majority. At the heart of his concern is the belief that we may not reasonably expect careful and honest weighing of values about health care when the allocation concerns only the poor and not everyone.

The way to answer theoretically driven suspicions about what is likely to happen is to look at the values actually reported from the community meetings and at the actual behavior of the legislature. Despite the bias in representation, the values expressed in the community meetings describe a set of concerns rooted in the participants' thoughts about what makes health care important to them. When carefully inspected, the list of values does not appear to be the work of a group of "haves" masking an uncaring and miserly attitude toward "have-nots." Rather, the community-meeting participants actually did as they were asked by identifying what they think makes health care an important benefit in and for the community. Given the content of the value statements, the burden of argument falls to those who, for theoretical reasons, believe that a largely middle-class group of American citizens could produce only a distorted expression of values if they knew that the values would be used to help determine what health care services would be made securely available to the poor.

The idea that the legislature cannot be trusted to look after the interests of the poor is an extension of this same theoretical orientation, blended with awareness of the record in recent years of decreasing governmental commitment to welfare programs. The political story in Oregon is surely a complicated one, but the fact is that the legislature did find a way to add significant new dollars to medicaid in the 1991–93 budget. It may be that the criticisms and the spotlight of public attention helped motivate the legislature to give adequate support to the medicaid budget, but, in fact, their behavior was not what the critics' theory predicted it would be. When reality contradicts what theory predicts, it is time to reconsider the theory.

A third concern focuses on a subset of the community—namely, health care providers—and urges that their basic ethic of patient advocacy will be corrupted if they play an active part in rationing health care.[23] As articulated by Robert Veatch in an earlier article, this argument holds that health care providers, particularly physicians, should never get into the business of rationing care, either at the bedside or at the statehouse through decisionmaking roles on commissions. In his view, physicians might be consultants to such a commission—the role played by those physicians on the expert panels that provided the HSC with outcome probability estimates—but they should not have been decisionmakers when allocation of resources is at stake. Physicians, Veatch argues, give great weight to consequences in their moral reasoning, making them too eager to pursue utilitarian cost-effectiveness goals to the detriment of moral considerations based on justice and rights.[24] Historically, Veatch's concern is rooted in the fact that the HSC first turned to cost-benefit analysis and a quantitative formula to conduct its prioritization task. However, despite Veatch's expectations about excessive utilitarianism on the part of a physician-dominated commission, the final list is primarily structured by a different moral logic that gives greater importance to values other than cost-effectiveness.[25] According to the commission report, the cost-benefit ratio has only a weak correlation with an item's position on the list.[26] The categories are dominant in explaining the priorities, and, as has been discussed, the method for ranking the categories was consciously influenced by a variety of values among which cost-effectiveness was included, but certainly not dominant.

A fourth concern asserts that the Oregon Plan, which requires considerable societal effort, amounts to a futile tinkering with a fundamentally defective system.[27] For these critics, the clear moral imperative is to get to a system of universal access to basic health care by the shortest possible path. Setting priorities is an intellectually and socially daunting exercise that merely postpones getting down to real business on the primary challenge: making a commitment to every citizen and seriously rooting out wasteful administrative and technical practices in the health care delivery system.

This concern is based partly on the belief that there is so much inefficiency in the U.S. health care system that capturing the revenues now wasted can easily provide enough resources to bring those currently uninsured into the system. The first response to this criticism is to assert that there is no intrinsic hostility in the Oregon Plan to the idea of improved efficiency; in fact, the laws call for movement in this direction. The second response, however, is more important. Both the Oregon Plan and the radical reform plan combine political and ethical judgments. Both strategies are committed to change the status quo in the direction of greater equity (and other important social values such as autonomy, efficiency, improved general welfare, and a higher common good). Most advocates of the Oregon Plan also call for more sweeping reforms. Most view the current laws as staging places for wider reforms. The Oregon Plan has brought a lethargic system into motion in Oregon. It is also doing something that sooner or later the advocates of sweeping reforms must face: how to differentiate among health services in relation to community values so that we can be sure that what is most important to the community is also most securely situated in the health care benefit packages guaranteed to the community.

A fifth moral concern is rooted in the technical difficulty of constructing a prioritized list of health services. On the one hand, critics argue that health care services are too complex to be prioritized with scientific validity.[28] Outcomes research is too slow and cumbersome to offer any hope for a scientifically based prioritization. Expert opinion ultimately may not be reliable because health care providers, the relevant experts, have a monetary interest in arranging for their typical services to score high on any prioritized list. On the other hand, information about the way people value specific services in the abstract, as opposed to when they actually need them, raises serious methodological problems. How these values can be validly and accurately discovered and then related to technical information about outcomes for specific services is thought by some to be an insurmountable obstacle. These theoretical considerations, it is urged, cast grave doubt on the prudence of attempting to base social policy on such questionable data. The answer to this concern, now that the list exists, is to inspect it to see whether it is the nonsensical product that the theorists predict. The critics have not analyzed the actual list. Their conviction that harm will come of its use still rests on their not fully disclosed rationales for slowly and painstakingly gathering an enormous amount of health services data before even thinking about setting priorities for allocating and managing society's collective investment in health care.

Meanwhile, the commission has made a good faith effort and produced a list that combines public values and expert opinion into a set of allocation priorities. Oregon legislators have taken the list and used it to focus debate, public testimony, and budgetary decisionmaking. They have found it a useful tool for actually expanding health care budget commitments to the poor of Oregon, and unless the program is derailed, the list's use will have moved Oregon forward in its much needed effort to bring aid to 450,000 Oregonians who are now uninsured for health care.

All of the aforementioned criticisms are an important feature of the ethical challenge entailed in the Oregon Plan. They have surely influenced the care, patience, and commitment with which the HSC went about producing the priority list. Concerns about fairness surely helped motivate the legislature to appropriate significant new dollars for the medicaid budget. In short, the criticisms have done just what they are supposed to do in an open democratic process—keep the plan moving in an ethically acceptable direction.

REFLECTIONS ON RATIONING AND COMMUNITY SOLIDARITY

At the heart of the ethical problem that the Oregon Plan seeks to address is the historical fact that our current system of solidarity for health care assigns some citizens the invidious status of *outsiders*. The history of the growth of third-party coverage since World War II reveals a public policy tending toward universal entitlement but lacking clear public commitment to the value of social solidarity on which such an entitlement logically rests. Between 1940 and 1950 the proportion of the population with employment-based hospital insurance increased from 9 percent to 57 percent.[29] By the early 1970s, after the passage of medicare and medicaid, the proportion of the people under age 65 with some form of third-party support for health care reached approximately 80 percent[30] and has hovered within 5 percentage points of that level to the present. Those without insurance are simply left outside the circle of solidarity that the majority enjoy.

Michael Walzer, in his analysis of the complex value of pluralism in contemporary society, offers instructive reflections on this point. He notes that the growth of communal provision of health care through both public and private third-party systems gives a historical validation to the desire for health care, which transforms the *desire* into a socially recognized *need*.[31] Once the desire is transformed into a socially validated need, the distributional logic for health care should relate to illness, not wealth. In such a society, to be deprived of access to health care is a double loss. Those left out of third-party solidarity suffer both the misfortune of illness and the insult of exclusion.

The mistaken use of wealth as the basis for health care distribution is perpetuated by society's failure to achieve full consciousness of the degree of solidarity implicit in all third-party financing arrangements. The community-meeting process organized by Oregon Health Decisions involved an effort to counteract society's lack of attentiveness to the structure and consequences of an unfinished commitment to third-party financing for health care. The community-meeting process functions as a vehicle for articulating moral discomfort with the fact that our current system of excluding some of our fellow citizens from the solidarity of third-party support contradicts fundamental values we publicly espouse. The capacity to exercise meaningful community responsibility for the institution of health care is especially needed now as the U.S. political community tackles its unfinished agenda of universal access, while simultaneously addressing legitimate concerns for cost containment and rational allocation of health care resources.

NOTES

1. Daniel Bell, *The Cultural Contradictions of Capitalism* (Basic Books, 1976), pp. 196–97.

2. Oregon Health Services Commission, *Prioritization of Health Services: A Report to the Governor and the Legislature* (Salem, 1991).

3. William B. Schwartz and Henry J. Aaron, "The Achilles Heel of Health Care Rationing," *New York Times*, July 9, 1990 (op-ed page).

4. See Arthur L. Caplan, "How Can We Deny Health Care to Poor While Others Get Face Lifts?" *Los Angeles Times*, April 25, 1989 (opinion page); and Tom Higgins, "Oregon Plan Doesn't Merit a Medicaid Waiver," *Healthweek*, May 21, 1990, p. 20.

5. Oregon Health Services Commission, *Prioritization of Health Services*, pp. 69–71.

6. Personal communication from Darren Coffman, Oregon Health Services Commission staff statistician.

7. Adapted from Oregon Health Services Commission, *Prioritization of Health Services*, appendix G, pp. 11–12.

8. Robert M. Kaplan and J. P. Anderson, "A General Health Policy Model: Update and Applications," *HSR: Health Services Research*, vol. 23 (June 1988), pp. 203–35.

9. Romana Hasnain and Michael Garland, "Health Care in Common: Report of the Oregon Health Decisions Community Meetings Process," Oregon Health Decisions, Portland, April 1990. The report is included in Oregon Health Services Commission, *Prioritization of Health Services*, appendix F. See also Michael J. Garland and Romana Hasnain, "Health Care in Common: Set-

ting Priorities in Oregon," *Hastings Center Report*, vol. 20 (September–October 1990), pp. 16–18.

10. Oregon Health Services Commission, *Prioritization of Health Services*, pp. 18–22 and appendix G.

11. Harvey D. Klevit and others, "Prioritization of Health Care Services: A Progress Report by the Health Services Commission," *Archives of Internal Medicine*, vol. 151 (May 1991), pp. 912–16.

12. Personal communication from Paige Sipes-Metzler, executive director of the Health Services Commission.

13. Norman Daniels, "Is the Oregon Rationing Plan Fair?" *Journal of the American Medical Association*, vol. 265 (May 1, 1991), pp. 2332–35.

14. Oregon Health Services Commission, *Prioritization of Health Services*, pp. 18–22 and appendix G.

15. Ibid., pp. 23–28 and appendix D.

16. Higgins, "Oregon Plan Doesn't Merit a Medicaid Waiver."

17. "Poor Children and Women Targeted for Medicaid Reductions in Oregon," *CDF Reports* (Children's Defense Fund), August 1990, pp. 1, 6–7; Virginia Morell, "Oregon Puts Bold Health Plan on Ice," *Science*, August 3, 1990, pp. 470–71; and Peter B. Budetti, "Medicaid Rationing in Oregon: Political Wolf in a Philosopher's Sheepskin," *Health Matrix: Case Western Reserve University Journal of Law Medicine* (forthcoming).

18. Daniels, "Is the Oregon Rationing Plan Fair?"

19. Leonard Fleck, "The Oregon Medicaid Experiment: Is It Just Enough?" *Business and Professional Ethics Journal*, vol. 9 (Fall–Winter 1990), pp. 201–17.

20. Daniels, "Is the Oregon Rationing Plan Fair?"

21. Caplan, "How Can We Deny Health Care to Poor?"

22. Daniels, "Is the Oregon Rationing Plan Fair?"

23. Robert M. Veatch, "Deciding Levels of Care: The Case for Public Control," paper read for a conference, Drawing the Line: Defining a Basic Level for Health Care, sponsored by the Center for Biomedical Ethics at the University of Minnesota, October 1990.

24. Robert M. Veatch, "Should Basic Care Get Priority? Doubts about Rationing the Oregon Way," *Kennedy Institute of Ethics Journal*, vol. 1 (September 1991), pp. 187–206.

25. Klevit and others, "Prioritization of Health Care Services."

26. Oregon Health Services Commission, *Prioritization of Health Services*, p. 28.

27. Arnold Relman, "The Trouble with Rationing," *New England Journal of Medicine*, vol. 323 (September 27, 1990), pp. 911–13; David U. Himmelstein and Steffie Woolhandler, "Cost without Benefit: Administrative Waste in U.S. Health Care," *New England Journal of Medicine*, vol. 314 (February 13, 1986), pp. 441–45; and David U. Himmelstein and Steffie Woolhandler, "A National

Health Program for the United States: A Physicians' Proposal," *New England Journal of Medicine*, vol. 320 (January 12, 1989), pp. 102–08.

28. Schwartz and Aaron, "Achilles Heel of Health Care Rationing."

29. Odin W. Anderson, *Health Care Services in the United States: A Growth Enterprise since 1875* (Ann Arbor, Mich.: Health Administration Press, 1985), pp. 134, 142.

30. *National Health Insurance Resource Book*, Committee Print, House Committee on Ways and Means (Government Printing Office, 1974), p. 74.

31. Michael Walzer, *Spheres of Justice: A Defense of Pluralism and Equality* (Basic Books, 1983), pp. 86–91.

ROBERT M. KAPLAN

A Quality-of-Life Approach to Health Resource Allocation

Today's world is witness to a remarkable disparity in both health and health care. In general, westernized countries with modern health care systems achieve better outcomes according to traditional measures of life expectancy and infant mortality. Even within westernized countries, however, there is substantial variation in expenditure on health care and little evidence that these variations result in better health outcomes.[1] The primary challenge is to use resources in a way that will maximize benefits. Oregon's Senate Bill 27 addresses this problem by maximizing net health benefits within the constraints of limited resources.[2] Net benefits are defined as life-expectancy and quality-of-life improvements anticipated from the intervention minus the anticipated side effects or consequences of treatment. These are expressed as a combined index of life expectancy and quality of life. This paper focuses on the quantification of the health outcomes. Before presenting the model of health outcome, I consider the cost problem.

THE RESOURCE ALLOCATION PROBLEM

The United States spends more than $600 billion on health care each year. Estimates for 1991 range as high as $750 billion. This has been estimated to be about 12 percent of the gross national product, and it is projected that health care costs will double by 1995 and triple by the turn of the century. If these forecasts are accurate, the United States will spend more than 15 percent of its GNP on health care by the turn of the century.

High expenditures on health care have raised serious concerns about the likelihood that American products can successfully compete with those offered by foreign competitors. For example, the Chrysler Corporation spends about $700 per automobile on health care costs; the comparable figure for Japanese automakers is less than $300. Discrepancies in health insurance account for a large portion of the cost differences in making products in various countries. In 1986 Great Britain spent only about 6 percent of its GNP on health care, and West Germany spent only about 8 percent. If these discrepancies continue, American products will probably fail in international competitions, and the balance of trade will possibly become even more severely distorted. Ultimately, the consequences for the United States economy could be very serious.

Arnold Relman suggested that there are three basic deficiencies in our health care system.[3] The first is that health care costs too much. Those who pay for health care, primarily large employers and governments, can no longer afford to continue offering the same level of services. A second problem is that our system is inequitable. Even though we spend more on health care as a proportion of the GNP than any other country does, we still have between 35 and 40 million people who have either no insurance or inadequate resources to cover care. The third, and perhaps most challenging, problem is that we have failed to be good consumers of health care. Theoretically, we purchase health care to obtain health. Yet, we know very little about the relationship between care and health outcome. Many of the services we purchase may be either unnecessary or ineffective.[4] Health care is the only major industry in the United States that does not account for what it produces. To help resolve these problems, we need models that consider the costs and the effects of health care.

Cost-Utility Analysis

There probably will never be enough health care resources to satisfy all of society's needs. Cost-utility analysis and other decision models are useful in helping to decide between competing alternatives. Economic models do not simply deal with costs. Formal economic and decision analyses consider outputs—the goods and services that society values. Exercises, such as the one conducted by the Oregon Health Services Commission, require that the output of any given service be evaluated. In such analyses, independent assessments of different services are of little value. The only way to compare competing alternatives is to express the output of various services in a common metric. The difficulty is that the objectives of different services in health care are typically measured in different outcome units.

Some critics have suggested that decision analysis cannot be conducted, because it is like comparing apples and oranges. We argue that, in fact, most allocation decisions do require choices between apples and oranges. For example, treatments have benefits and they have side effects. Treatments have effects on various outcomes, and medical experiments usually produce profiles of different outcomes. A treatment may reduce pain while increasing gastrointestinal disturbance. Effective cancer therapy causes severe nausea and vomiting. Ultimately, we must make a decision about whether the treatment should be used or whether it should be avoided. Cost-utility analysis places all outcomes in a common unit. The method for achieving this will be described shortly. First, however, it will be necessary to separate cost-utility from cost-effectiveness and cost-benefit analysis.

Definition of Terms

The terms *cost-utility*, *cost-effectiveness*, and *cost-benefit* are used inconsistently in the medical literature.[5] Some economists have favored the assessment of cost-benefit. These approaches measure both program costs and treatment outcomes in dollar units. For example, treatment outcomes are evaluated in relation to changes in cost of medical services, economic productivity, and so forth. Treatments are cost-beneficial if the economic return exceeds treatment costs. Diabetic patients who are aggressively treated, for example, may need fewer medical services. The savings associated with decreased services might exceed treatment costs. As argued by Louise Russell, the requirement that health care treatments reduce costs may be unrealistic.[6] Patients are willing to pay for improvements in health status just as they are willing to pay for other desirable goods and services. We do not treat cancer to save money. Instead, treatments are given to achieve better health outcomes.

Cost-effectiveness is an alternative approach in which the unit of outcome is a health or treatment effect. In recent years, cost-effectiveness has gained considerable attention. Some approaches, such as those advocated by B. T. Yates and Nancy DeMuth, emphasize simple, treatment-specific outcomes.[7] For example, Yates considers the cost per pound lost as a measure of cost-effectiveness of weight-loss programs. The major difficulty with cost-effectiveness methodologies is that they do not allow for comparison across very different treatment interventions. Weight-loss programs evaluated in terms of cost per pound lost cannot be compared with blood pressure reduction programs evaluated in terms of cost per millimeter of mercury reduced. Health care administrators often need to choose between investments in very different alternatives. They may need to decide between supporting liver transplantation for a few patients and prenatal counseling for numerous patients. For the same cost, they may achieve a large effect for a few people or a small effect for a large number of people. The treatment-specific outcomes used in cost-effectiveness studies do not permit these comparisons.

Cost-utility approaches use the expressed preference or utility of a treatment effect as the unit of outcome. As noted in World Health Organization documents, the goals of health care are to add years to life and life to years.[8] In other words, health care is designed to make people live longer (increase the life expectancy) and to have higher quality of lives in the years before death. Cost-utility studies use outcome measures that combine mortality outcomes with quality-of-life measurements. The utilities are the expressed preferences for observable states of function on a continuum bounded by 0.0 for death and 1.0 for optimum function.[9] In recent years, cost-utility approaches have gained increasing acceptance as methods for comparing many diverse options in health care.[10]

COMPARISONS ACROSS DIAGNOSES: THE INCREMENTAL OUTCOME PROBLEM

To resolve health care cost problems, formal decisionmaking models are needed. Mathematical models of decisionmaking are now being proposed in many health care systems. For example, these models have been suggested for use in European, Australian, and American health care systems. There is a growing recognition that health care resources are very limited. The British National Health Service, for example, has recognized the need to prioritize competing demands on their very limited budgets.[11] Yet, prioritization schemes make little sense without some consideration of outcome.

The most important challenge in developing a formal model for re-source allocation is in defining a common unit of health benefit. Typically, the value of each specific intervention in health care is de-termined by considering a measure specific to the intervention or the disease process. Treatments for hypertension, for example, are evaluated in terms of blood pressure, while those for diabetes are evaluated by blood glucose. Yet, it is difficult to determine the relative value of investing in blood glucose rather than in blood pressure re-duction. Traditional public health measures, such as life expectancy, are usually too crude to allow appropriate prioritization. I believe, however, that a general model of health outcome is both feasible and practical.

A GENERAL HEALTH POLICY MODEL

To understand health outcomes, it is necessary to build a comprehen-sive theoretical model of health status. This model includes several components. The main aspects of the model are mortality (death) and morbidity (health-related quality of life). Several papers in this vol-ume suggest that diseases and disabilities are important for two rea-sons—illness may cause the life expectancy to be shortened, and ill-ness may make life less desirable at times before death (health-related quality of life).[12]

During the last two decades, a group of investigators at the Univer-sity of California, San Diego, has developed a general health policy model (GHPM). Central to the model is a general conceptualization of health status. The model separates aspects of health status into dis-tinct components: life expectancy (mortality), functioning and symp-toms (morbidity), preference for observed functional states (utility), and duration of stay in health states (prognosis).

Mortality

A model of health outcomes necessarily includes a component for mortality. Indeed, many public health statistics focus exclusively on mortality through estimations of crude mortality rates, age-adjusted mortality rates, and infant mortality rates. Death is an important outcome that must be included in any comprehensive conceptualization of health.

Morbidity

Besides death, behavioral dysfunction is also an important outcome. The GHPM considers functioning in three areas: mobility, physical activity, and social activity. Descriptions of the measures of these aspects of function are given in many different publications.[13] Most public health indicators are relatively insensitive to variations toward the well end of the continuum. Measures of infant mortality, to give an extreme example, ignore all people capable of reading this article, since they have lived for more than one year after their births (I assume that no infants are reading the article). Disability measures often ignore those in relatively well states. For example, the Rand Health Insurance Study reported that about 80 percent of the general population has no dysfunction. Thus, they would estimate that 80 percent of the population is well. Our method asks about symptoms or problems in addition to behavioral dysfunction.[14] In these studies, only about 12 percent of the general population reports no symptoms on a particular day. In other words, health symptoms or problems are a very common aspect of the human experience. Some might argue that symptoms are unimportant because they are subjective and unobservable. However, symptoms are highly correlated with the demand for medical services, expenditures on health care, and motivations to alter life-styles. Thus, we feel that the quantification of symptoms is very important.

Utility (Relative Importance)

Since various components of morbidity and mortality can be tabulated, it is important to consider their relative importance. For example, it is possible to develop measures that detect very minor symptoms. Yet, that these symptoms are measurable does not necessarily mean they are important. A patient may experience side effects but be willing to tolerate them because they are less important than the probable benefit that would be obtained if the medication was consumed. Not all outcomes are equally important. A treatment in which twenty of one hundred patients die is not equivalent to one in which twenty of one hundred patients develop nausea. An important component of the GHPM attempts to scale the various health outcomes according to their relative importance. In the preceding example, the relative importance of dying would be weighted more than developing nausea. The weighting is accomplished by rating all states on a continuum ranging from o.o (for dead) to 1.o (for optimum functioning). These ratings are typically provided by independent judges who are representative of the general population. Using this system, one can express the relative importance of states in relation to the life-death continuum. A point halfway on the scale (o.5) is regarded as halfway between optimum function and death. The weighting system has been described in several different publications.[15]

Prognosis

Another dimension of health status is the duration of a condition. A headache that lasts one hour is not equivalent to a headache that lasts one month. A cough that lasts three days is not equivalent to a cough that lasts three years. In considering the severity of illness, duration of the problem is central. As basic as this concept is, most contemporary models of health outcome measurement completely disregard the duration component. In the GHPM, the term *prognosis* refers to the probability of transition among health states over the course of time. Besides considering the duration of problems, the model considers the point at which the problem begins. A person may have no symptoms or dysfunctions currently but may have a high probability of health problems in the future. The prognosis component of the model takes these transitions into consideration and applies a discount rate for events that occur in the future. The quality-of-well-being scale (QWB) is a method for estimating some components of the general model. The QWB questionnaire categorizes individuals according to functioning and symptoms. Other components of the model are obtained from other data sources.[16]

A mathematical formula integrates components of the model to express outcomes in a common measurement unit. Using information on current functioning and duration, one can express the health outcomes in terms of equivalents of well-years of life or, as some have described them, quality-adjusted life-years (QALYs). The model for point-in-time QWB is

$QWB = 1 - $ (*observed morbidity* × *morbidity weight*)
     $-$ (*observed physical activity* × *physical activity weight*)
     $-$ (*observed social activity* × *social activity weight*)
     $-$ (*observed symptom/problem* × *symptom/problem weight*).

The net cost-utility ratio is defined as

$$\frac{net\ cost}{net\ QWB \times \ duration\ in\ years} = \frac{cost\ of\ treatment\ -\ cost\ of\ alternative}{(QWB\ treatment\ -\ QWB\ alternative) \times\ duration\ in\ years}.$$

 Consider, for example, a person who is in an objective state of functioning that is rated by community peers as 0.5 on a 0.0 to 1.0 scale. If the person remains in the state for one year, he or she has lost the equivalent of one-half year of life. So, for example, a person of limited mobility, who requires a cane or walker to get around the community, might be hypothetically at 0.5. Over the course of an entire year, he or she would lose the equivalent of one year of life. A person who has the flu may also get 0.5, but the illness might last only three days. Thus, the total loss in well-years might be $3/365 \times 0.5 = 0.004$ well-years.

How This Model Differs from Traditional Conceptualizations

 The two main differences between the GHPM and other approaches to health outcome measurement are the attempt to express benefits and consequences of health in a common unit known as the well-year or quality-adjusted life-year, and the emphasis on "the area under the curve" rather than point-in-time measurement. In the following sections, I argue that the general approach to health outcome is, intuitively, what patients and consumers use as a guide. Their physicians may be more directed by a less comprehensive model that considers only a component of health outcome. For example, health care providers might focus on a component of health outcome such as blood pressure. Focusing on blood pressure might allow the provider to disregard all the other effects blood pressure management has on health outcome. Consumers must integrate various sources of information in their decision process. They are intuitively directed toward maximization of health outcomes. At times these decisions become overwhelming, however, and the use of a formal model may help them to make decisions.

A basic objective for most people is to function without symptoms as long as possible. Clearly, early death contradicts this objective. Illness and disability during the interval between birth and death also reduce the total potential health status during a lifetime. Many approaches to health assessment consider only current functioning, snapshots of health status known as point-in-time measures. The GHPM considers outcome throughout the life cycle, that is, the area under the curve. The more wellness a person experiences throughout the life span, the greater is the area under the curve. The success of interventions is marked by an expanded area.

The general nature of the GHPM leads to some conclusions that are different from more traditional medical approaches. For example, the traditional medical model focuses on specific diseases and on pathophysiology. Characteristics of illness are quantified according to blood chemistry or in relation to problems in a specific organ system. Often, the conclusions reached by focusing on disease-specific outcome measures are different from those reached by using a more general outcome measure. For example, studies on the reduction of blood cholesterol have demonstrated reductions in deaths resulting from coronary heart disease. The same studies, however, have failed to demonstrate reductions in total deaths from all causes combined.[17] All studies in the published literature in which patients are assigned to cholesterol-lowering through diet or medication, or to a control group, have revealed that reductions in cardiovascular mortality for those in the cholesterol-lowering group are compensated for by increases in mortality from other causes.[18] A meta-analysis of these studies has demonstrated that the average statistical difference for increase in deaths from non-illness causes (that is, accidents, murders, and so forth) is larger than the average statistical difference for reduction in cardiovascular deaths.[19]

Similar results have been reported for reductions in cardiovascular deaths attributable to taking aspirin. The disease-specific approach focuses on deaths due to myocardial infarction because there is a biological model to describe the reason that aspirin use should reduce heart attacks. Yet, in a controlled experiment in which physician subjects were randomly assigned to take aspirin or a placebo, there was no difference in total deaths between the two groups.[20] Aspirin may reduce the chances of dying from a myocardial infarction, but it does not reduce the chance of dying.[21] The traditional, diagnosis-specific medical model argues that there is a benefit in aspirin because it reduces heart attack, but the general health policy model argues that there is no benefit in aspirin because there is no change in the chances of dying from all causes.[22]

This same line of reasoning applies to many other areas of health care. Many treatments produce benefits for a specific outcome but induce side effects that are often neglected in the analysis. Estimates of the benefits of surgery must take into consideration the fact that surgery causes dysfunction through wounds that must heal before any realization of the treatment benefits. Further, surgeries often create complications. The general approach to health status assessment attempts to gain a global picture of the net treatment benefits, taking into consideration both treatment benefits, side effects, and estimates of their relative importance.

APPLICATION OF THE MODEL TO PROBLEMS OF HEALTH RESOURCE ALLOCATION

The general health policy model has now been used in a variety of different settings. Some of these will be reviewed briefly below.

Oregon Bill 27

Perhaps the best proposal to use a resource allocation model in the United States is currently under consideration in Oregon. In 1989 the Oregon State Senate passed Senate Bill 27, creating the Oregon Health Services Commission, which was given the task of prioritizing various services reimbursed by the Oregon medicaid program. The first step in this process was to hold a series of public hearings during which 1,700 people testified at forty-seven town meetings. This group came up with thirteen basic values such as prevention, quality of life, cost-effectiveness, and equity. Then the quality-of-well-being scale was used to estimate the effectiveness of many services. Input was obtained from forty-five specialty groups to determine what effects various treatments produced. The Oregon commission did not want to use weights obtained from the state of California. Instead, it performed its own scaling studies to obtain Oregon weights. Except in three cases, however, these weights were similar to those from California. In an initial phase, costs were also estimated for procedures, and a prioritization list was created. But a later version of the list released in February 1991 allowed for adjustments according to the thirteen values identified in the town meetings. Essentially, this process permitted the commission to reprioritize procedures according to the thirteen basic values. Ultimately, the commission produced a list of 709 condition-treatment pairs. In June 1991 the funding line was drawn at condition-treatment pair 587.

One of the significant issues in the Oregon exercise is the decision by the commission to use its intuition in ranking the cost-utility of services. The GHPM calls for a rank ordering based on cost per well-year gained. In the initial exercise, the Oregon Health Services Commission considered the rank ordering of numerous procedures. When the list was completed, it was concluded that many of the rankings were counterintuitive. The commission was clearly bothered by these findings. The reason that the outcomes were counterintuitive, however, had more to do with the data sources than with the methods. Poorly or hastily conducted analyses will lead to counterintuitive rankings. The commission was under unusual time pressure to produce cost-utility ratios for an enormous number of procedures, whereas careful analysis might have taken several decades. The problem was that the commission either seriously overestimated or seriously underestimated the value of some services. Careful reanalysis would almost certainly rectify the problem. Instead, the commission chose to subjectively rerank procedures. In fact, it might be argued that the new rankings are counterintuitive because many of the highly ranked procedures apparently have little or no health benefit. There is concern that political considerations, rather than data, allowed the realignment of some services.

David Hadorn interpreted the reassessment of priorities as a rejection of the GHPM.[23] Part of his criticism was that high-benefit–high-cost procedures come out the same as low-cost–low-benefit procedures. Yet, this result is not necessarily counterintuitive. The capacity to help a large number of people gain a small amount of health status may equal the capacity to produce a big difference for a small number of people. Indeed, it was this type of allocation problem the model was designed to solve. Hadorn's principal concern was that some extremely expensive, but potentially helpful, procedures might not be funded. Spending huge sums of money to potentially save a life is described by Hadorn as "the rule of rescue." He argues that there is a sympathetic motivation to engage in rescue. A reanalysis of the Oregon rankings, however, may address Hadorn's concerns. When done properly, the system favors funding of virtually all services that produce benefit. But if a service is extremely expensive, it also must be very effective. It is possible that some lifesaving services may not be funded. By not funding these extremely expensive services for very few people, however, revenues are generated to fund services for other people. All things considered, the GHPM produces more health for more people. The rule of rescue condemns large numbers of people who might achieve a small benefit from the services to going without. No decision is easy, but the system attempts to optimize health benefits.

Another ethical argument against the GHPM is that the metric should not be linear. Other things being equal, improvements for those who are sick should be valued more than improvements for those who are nearly well. Thus, improvements in health status from 0.3 to 0.6 should be valued more than those from 0.7 to 1.0. This is consistent with some theories of distributive justice.[24] If this argument is correct, however, judges should see the value of improving health status for sick people as greater than the value of improving health status for well people. Yet, this is not confirmed by data from judgment studies.

The preferences for the states for the general health policy model do come from community judgment. Indeed, the difference between 0.3 and 0.6 is defined to be equal to the difference between 0.7 and 1.0. Further, sick and well people judge these cases similarly. The benefits of helping to cure very sick people are explicitly part of the model. Consider, for instance, treatments that produce complete cures. For those who initially have low values, the potential for benefit is very great; for those who are nearly well, the potential for benefit is smaller. For example, the difference between 0.4 and 1.0 is 0.6, while the difference between 0.9 and 1.0 is 0.1. Curing one person who begins at 0.4 is equal to curing 6 people beginning at 0.9.

The original Oregon exercise provides one example of how a prioritization scheme might be implemented. Unfortunately, the Health Services Commission gave up the part of the model that maximized benefits in favor of a more subjective system. I will return to some of the difficulties in using the system later.

The EuroQol Group

A similar approach has been taken by a group of investigators in Europe. This group includes researchers and analysts at the Health Economics Research Group at Brunell University; the Academy of Finland; the National Public Health Institute; the University of Helsinki; the Swedish Institute for Health Economics; the National Institute of Public Health of Norway; the Department of Academic Psychiatry, Middlesex; the University of London; Erasmus University in Rotterdam; the Dutch Institute of Medical Technology Assessment; the departments of Economics, Law, and Public Health and Social Medicine of the University of Rotterdam; and the Centre for Health Economics at the University of York.

The purpose of the EuroQol group is to develop standardized non-disease-specific outcome measures similar to the general health policy model. Conceptually, the approaches are very similar, though the exact methodologies differ. In particular, the EuroQol rating classifications do not include symptoms but do include pain and anxiety. In addition, the method for obtaining the utility weightings is different. Early work in the EuroQol group suggests that there are striking similarities in weights obtained from subjects in different European communities. Thus far, preference studies have been conducted in England, the Netherlands, and Sweden. My calculations suggest that these weights are also similar to those obtained in California and in Oregon. Although there are methodological differences, it is of interest that a conceptually similar methodology is emerging in different parts of the industrialized world.[25] These results suggest that obtaining reliable utility weights is feasible.

METHODOLOGICAL ISSUES

Despite the important contribution of the Oregon exercise, many methodological issues remain unresolved. A serious failure of the Oregon analysis is that it generated a large list of cost-utility ratios in too short a period. In some cases the data source underlying the analysis was much stronger than in others. Indeed, clinical judgment served as one of the most important sources of information for the overall analysis. The hasty evaluation of many services probably led to many inaccurate representations of treatment effectiveness, which may have led commissioners to incorrectly reject the model when they should have questioned the analysis. As the field of cost-utility analysis progresses, it will be important to evaluate the data sources carefully.

Groups in different parts of the world have suggested standards for cost-utility analysis. For example, standards for economic analyses for the evaluation of pharmaceutical products have been proposed in Australia; similar standards have been proposed for international studies and in the United Kingdom.[26] Recommendations for standardized quality-of-life measurement in Europe have also been suggested.[27]

Michael Drummond and his associates raised ten questions about cost-utility analyses.[28] For example, they asked whether a well-defined question was posed in answerable form (issue 1). They questioned whether the treatment was well defined in comparison with alternative treatments (issue 2). A related concern is how the proof of effectiveness was established (issue 3). Was it based on hard evidence from a randomized trial? When randomized trials were used, were the selection criteria so restrictive that the results are not generalizable? Each of these concerns must be considered in the Oregon prioritization scheme. In Oregon the estimates of effectiveness came primarily from clinical judgment and rarely from clinical trials. There is some concern that clinicians might engage in "gaming" to enhance their specialty or may naively overestimate the clinical impact of their procedures.

A fourth issue was whether all relevant costs and consequences were identified for each alternative. Cost-utility analysis requires that the appropriate resources required to produce the outcome were valued (issue 5). Another question is how the consequences of treatment were valued and whether they were even measured. The timing of treatment must also be considered. Some treatments require the use of current resources to produce future gains (issue 6). Such analyses require discounting, because current resources could have been used for alternative purposes (issue 7). The pricing of services in Oregon were made public with the release of the actuary report on May 1, 1991.

An eighth issue was whether incremental analysis was performed. In other words, did the analysis consider the difference in the effects of two alternative treatments and the differences in costs? One criticism of the Oregon exercise is that it looked at incremental benefits but did not use incremental costs. A ninth issue concerns sensitivity analysis. Sensitivity analysis must consider the "softness" of the information used to estimate costs and effects. This is typically done by assuming the best case and the worst case. For instance, the analysts might assume that the treatment is half as effective as in the base-case analysis or twice as effective. The analysis is then rerun to determine whether the conclusions change with these variations. The Oregon analysis might benefit from sensitivity analyses, particularly for procedures near the cutoff line.

Unfortunately, we still have very little understanding of the statistical properties underlying cost-utility ratios (issue 9). For example, the variability of the ratio will be larger than the variability of the numerator or the denominator. Most analyses use point estimates for the ratios and confidence intervals are rarely reported. Finally, it is important that we consider how cost-utility ratios will be used (issue 10). There is a tendency for numbers resulting from these analyses to have a life of their own. We must recognize that the cost-utility ratios are estimates. Various analyses should identify where the data are weak and where more investigation is required. Analyses, such as those conducted in Oregon, should undergo continual scrutiny and the numbers should undergo continual reevaluation.

SUMMARY AND CONCLUSION

A GHPM is proposed for determining appropriate resource allocation. It is important to emphasize that cost-utility models are imprecise and have only recently been given serious consideration in health policy debates. We need considerably more data to make informed decisions in the future.

The application of the model by the Oregon Health Services Commission should be applauded. However, the commission rushed the analysis and apparently made many errors in estimating treatment benefit, so that the prioritization list appears counterintuitive. In response, the commission rejected the model in favor of a more subjective scheme. As a result, the final Oregon Plan may fail to realize the promise of producing the most benefit for the most people. Had the commission carefully reviewed the analysis, it might have identified the reasons some rankings seemed counterintuitive.

Applications of these models should be considered an iterative process. Analyses will identify weaknesses in the data. These should stimulate new studies and redevelopment of the models. Models and analyses do currently exist, however, and it is not premature to begin applying these in the resource allocation process.

NOTES

1. John E. Wennberg, "Small Area Analysis in the Medical Care Outcome Problem," in Lee B. Sechrest, Edward Perrin, and John P. Bunder, eds., *Research Methodology: Strengthening Causal Interpretations of Nonexperimental Data* (Beverly Hills: Sage, 1990).

2. David C. Hadorn, "Defining Basic Health Benefits Using Clinical Guidelines: A Model Proposal for Discussion," paper prepared for PERS conference, Sacramento, Calif., April 1991.

3. Sandra Hackman and Robert Howard, "Confronting the Crisis in Health Care: An Interview with Arnold Relman," *Technology Review*, vol. 92 (July 1989), pp. 30–40.

4. Robert H. Brook and Kathleen N. Lohr, "Will We Need to Ration Effective Health Care?" *Issues in Science and Technology*, vol. 3 (Fall 1986), pp. 68–77.

5. Peter Doubilet, Milton C. Weinstein, and Barbara J. McNeil, "Use and Misuse of the Term 'Cost Effective' in Medicine," *New England Journal of Medicine*, vol. 314 (January 23, 1986), pp. 253–56.

6. Louise B. Russell, *Is Prevention Better Than Cure?* (Brookings, 1986).

7. B. T. Yates and Nancy M. DeMuth, "Alternative Funding and Incentive Mechanisms for Health Systems," in Anthony Broskowski, Edward S. Marks, and Simon H. Budman, eds., *Linking Health and Mental Health* (Beverly Hills: Sage, 1981), pp. 77–99.

8. Robert M. Kaplan and James W. Bush, "Health-Related Quality of Life Measurement for Evaluation Research and Policy Analysis," *Health Psychology*, vol. 1 (1982), pp. 61–80.

9. Ibid.; and World Health Organization, *Health Promotion: A Discussion Document on the Concept and Principles* (Copenhagen: World Health Organization

Regional Office for Europe, 1984); Robert M. Kaplan, "Human Preference Measurement for Health Decisions and the Evaluation of Long-Term Care," in Robert L. Kane and Rosalie A. Kane, eds., *Values and Long-Term Care* (Lexington, Mass.: Lexington Books, 1982), pp. 157–88; Robert M. Kaplan, "Behavior As a Central Outcome in Health Care," *American Psychologist*, vol. 45, no. 11 (1990), pp. 1211–20; and Robert M. Kaplan and John P. Anderson, "A General Health Policy Model: Update and Applications," *Health Services Research*, vol. 23 (June 1988), pp. 203–35.

10. Russell, *Is Prevention Better Than Cure?*; Milton C. Weinstein and William B. Stason, "Foundations of Cost-Effectiveness Analysis for Health and Medical Practice," *New England Journal of Medicine*, vol. 296 (March 31, 1977), pp. 716–21; and Alan Williams, "The Importance of Quality of Life in Policy Decisions," in Stuart R. Walker and Rachel M. Rosser, eds., *Quality of Life: Assessment and Application* (Boston: MTP Press, 1988), pp. 279–90.

11. Alan Maynard, "Economic Aspects in HIV Management," in Alan Maynard, ed., *Economic Aspects in HIV Management*, International Seminar Series: The Management of HIV Infection (London: Colwood Press, forthcoming).

12. Kaplan and Anderson, "General Health Policy Model: Update"; and Robert M. Kaplan and John P. Anderson, "The General Health Policy Model: An Integrated Approach," in Bert Spilker, ed., *Quality of Life Assessment in Clinical Trials* (Raven Press, 1990), pp. 131–49.

13. For summaries, see ibid.

14. Kaplan and Anderson, "General Health Policy Model: Integrated Approach."

15. Kaplan, "Human Preference Measurement"; Robert M. Kaplan, James W. Bush, and Charles C. Berry, "Health Status: Types of Validity and the Index of Well-Being," *Health Services Research*, vol. 11 (Winter 1976), pp. 478–507; Robert M. Kaplan, James W. Bush, and Charles C. Berry, "The Reliability, Stability, and Generalizability of a Health Status Index," in American Statistical Association, *Proceedings of the Social Status Section* (1978), pp. 704–09; and Robert M. Kaplan, James W. Bush, and Charles C. Berry, "Health Status Index: Category Rating versus Magnitude Estimation for Measuring Levels of Well-Being," *Medical Care*, vol. 17 (May 1979), pp. 501–25.

16. Kaplan and Anderson, "General Health Policy Model: Integrated Approach."

17. Lipid Research Clinics Program, "The Lipid Research Clinics Coronary Primary Prevention Trial Results: 1. Reduction in Incidence in Coronary Heart Disease," *Journal of the American Medical Association*, vol. 251 (January 20, 1984), pp. 351–64.

18. Robert M. Kaplan, "The Connection between Clinical Health Promotion and Health Status: A Critical Overview," *American Psychologist*, vol. 39, no. 7 (1984), pp. 755–65; and Robert M. Kaplan, "Behavioral Epidemiology, Health Promotion, and Health Services," *Medical Care*, vol. 23 (May 1985), pp. 564–83.

19. Matthew F. Mauldoon, Stephen B. Manuck, and Karen A. Matthews, "Effects of Cholesterol Lowering on Mortality: A Quantitative Review of Primary Prevention Trials," paper presented at the annual meeting of the American Psychological Association, Boston, August 1990.

20. R. M. Kaplan, "Health Outcome Models for Policy Analysis," *Health Psychology*, vol. 8, no. 6 (1989), pp. 723– 35.

21. Steering Committee of the Physicians' Health Study Research Group, "Preliminary Report: Findings from the Aspirin Component of the Ongoing Physicians' Health Study," *New England Journal of Medicine*, vol. 318 (January 28, 1988), pp. 262–64; and Steering Committee of the Physicians' Health Study Research Group, "Final Report on the Aspirin Component of the Ongoing Physicians' Health Study," *New England Journal of Medicine*, vol. 321 (July 20, 1989), pp. 129–35.

22. Maynard, "Economic Aspects in HIV Management."

23. David C. Hadorn, "Setting Health Care Priorities in Oregon: Cost-Effectiveness Meets the Rule of Rescue," *Journal of the American Medical Association*, vol. 265 (May 1, 1991), pp. 2218–25.

24. See Robert Veatch's paper in this volume.

25. EuroQol Group, "EuroQol—A New Facility for the Measurement of Health-Related Quality of Life," *Health Policy*, vol. 16 (1990), pp. 199–208.

26. David Evans and others, "The Use of Economic Analyses as a Basis of Inclusion of Pharmaceutical Products on Pharmaceutical Benefit Schemes," proposal to Australian Govenment, 1991; M. Drummond and others, "Standardizing Economic Evaluation Methodologies in Health Care: Practice, Problems, and Potential," in R. A. Luce and A. Elexhause, eds., *Standards for Socio-Economic Evaluation of Health Care Products and Services* (New York: Springer-Verlag 1990); and Michael F. Drummond, Greg Stoddard, and George W. Torrance, *Methods for the Economic Evaluation of Health Care Programmes* (Oxford University Press, 1987).

27. EuroQol Group, "EuroQol."

28. Drummond and others, "Standardizing Economic Evaluation Methodologies," and *Methods for Economic Evaluation*.

ROBERT M. VEATCH

The Oregon Experiment: Needless and Real Worries

The Oregon experiment in rationing health care for some medicaid recipients provides a long-awaited, desperately needed attempt to do something serious about our moral priorities for health care. As with any social experiment that really may have some effect, the Oregon effort is beginning to stimulate heated public policy debate. I have, from the beginning, been an enthusiastic supporter of the effort. Given the unfairness and inefficiency of the status quo, Americans can ill afford not to take some risk in trying serious alternatives. Nevertheless, at this point in the discussion, I believe that most is to be gained by examining the potential objections and trying to distinguish needless or false worries from those that should give real concern. I first raise three seemingly misplaced concerns and then discuss three problems that appear to pose real, serious threats unless significant changes are made in the way the plan operates. My conclusion is that the experiment is well worth trying—indeed, morally imperative—but that certain elements of the approach will do serious moral harm if they are not corrected.

THREE SURMOUNTABLE WORRIES

First, I should note three arguments surfacing against the Oregon experiment that are, to my way of thinking, misguided or, at the very least, reflect problems that are surmountable. These arguments come from different quarters—from the most conservative defenders of traditional medical practice, from romantics who oppose all rationalization and systemization, and from radicals who favor rationing, but only if applied to the wealthy.

The "No Need to Ration" Argument

The first false concern is voiced by those who claim there is no need to ration—that in a country as wealthy as ours we would have enough resources to do all the medical good we desired, if only. . . . At this point, some agenda completes the sentence which involves eliminating waste both within the health care system (abolishing useless defensive medicine and profit-driven useless procedures) and outside it (defense department expenditures, tobacco subsidies, or congressional junkets).

Those who offer this criticism misunderstand the nature of the problem. Even if all waste were eliminated (a utopian dream), there would still be countless medical procedures that would be truly beneficial for people—enough to consume the entire gross national product. Even more important, providing additional medical resources for a problem sometimes produces declining marginal utility. Just before one reaches the point where additional resources will do no more good, there is a point where additional resources will provide a very small, very inefficient increment of benefit. In a world of finite resources, it is irrational for a society to support a health plan that would do what is literally medically best for patients, when cutting slightly below that point would release resources to be used in ways that were much more efficient or equitable. Rational people will insist that their health care insurance not fund every possible medical benefit for them. Rationing at the point of deciding what insurance should cover is inevitable; it already happens in every insurance policy that has any coverage limits.[1]

"Quantification Is Repulsive" Argument

A second concern raised by critics is that the quantification of impossibly complex and subtle medical decisions necessitated by the Oregon experiment is either repulsive or misleading. It requires making crude simplifications, quantifying such harms as suffering, separation, and psychological deficits, and otherwise reducing complex, subjective judgments to computer-manipulated quantities.

It would be a mistake to underestimate the subtlety of the judgments. Yet, the problem is, in principle, no different from that of the clinician at the bedside who must make rough estimates of the benefits and harms of alternative courses of action. There is every reason to believe that more deliberate, more public, more complex number crunching is more reliable than casual, ad hoc, private guesses at the benefits and harms of alternatives. The use of the quality-of-well-being (QWB) index,[2] or some similar quality-adjusted life-year (QALY) approach,[3] is superior in public planning than an intuitive, subjective basis for decisions. The Oregon people should not be faulted for trying to quantify.

"Injustice of Targeting the Poor" Argument

The third argument heard against the Oregon experiment is one that is difficult to label unjustified. Many criticize targeting medicaid patients as the guinea pigs—and targeting one specific, vulnerable group of women and children at that.[4] They are right that it would be far better to develop a rationing plan in the context of a national, single-payer insurance system or universal insurance system.[5] Anyone engaged in the debate over the Basic Health Services Program is morally obliged to take part simultaneously in efforts to expand its application to a universal system of insurance. The need to make a health insurance system ethically responsible, however, is independent of the question of to whom it applies. The task of developing a morally defensible, equitable ranking system is just as great whether people can be convinced to apply it to all insurance or only to some aspects of medicaid. The funds available may be being used irresponsibly and inequitably. Continuing the project of deciding what is a fair use of funds must go on while the effort to include all health care in the system proceeds.

THREE REAL CONCERNS

Whereas these three commonly heard objections to the Oregon experiment may be overcome if dealt with carefully, there are three less obvious problems that, to me, are real concerns. They arise not because of the fact that Oregon has undertaken the project of trying to determine which health care is morally the highest priority but because of the specific assumptions and methods used.

Equivocation with the Concept of "Basic"

The use of the term *basic* to describe the health care that will receive priority in Oregon's rationing scheme is equivocal. From the beginning, *basic* has been used to refer to the care that would be funded under the Oregon effort. The legislation has been referred to as the Oregon Basic Health Services Act, the Oregon Health Decisions process continually referred to care that was basic, and one of the three "attributes" used by the Oregon Health Services Commission in ranking its "categories" of health care was whether it was "essential to basic health care."

The Health Services Commission makes clear that *basic*, by definition, has moral or public policy meaning: care is basic if it is within the level of services "below which it is felt no person should fall." Here *basic* is a synonym for *essential.*[6]

The problem is that at other times the term *basic* has an essentially nonmoral meaning. Care is basic if it is simple, low-tech, preventive, primary, and inexpensive, or is curative for acute conditions. The problem traces back to the pre–Coby Howard days,* when a judgment was made that so-called basic care, such as prenatal care and immunizations, should take priority over high-tech efforts to stave off dying through the use of organ and tissue transplants.

The equivocation in the use of the term *basic* permits the mistake of assuming that care that is nonmorally basic (simple, low-tech) is therefore morally basic (highest priority or most essential). The detail of the argument is virtually never stated. It must go something like the following.

Care that is nonmorally basic (simple, low-tech, inexpensive, preventive, or curative for acute illness) is the most cost-efficient care. The care that is the most cost-efficient is morally basic (the highest priority). Therefore, nonmorally basic care is morally basic as well.

When stated explicitly, the explanation of the term *basic* becomes problematic. It is a debatable, empirical claim whether nonmorally basic care is the most cost-efficient. For example, data would be needed

---

*Coby Howard, a young leukemia patient on medicaid, did not receive an expensive bone marrow transplant, because medicaid refused to pay for it. His subsequent death triggered the whole Oregon process.

to support the presumption that money spent on the thirty projected organ transplants for patients on medicaid would do less good than the same money spent on basic preventive care for three thousand people with no health insurance coverage.[7] Although that may be true, a large fraction of the transplant recipients will literally get a life-saving intervention, while many recipients of a basic preventive care package may see little or no benefit. I have no way of knowing which investment is the most cost-effective measured in QALYs added without seeing sophisticated empirical data.

Then, even if it is true that nonmorally basic care is more cost-efficient, it does not follow that it has a morally higher priority. Most moral systems incorporate criteria of moral right-making that extend beyond the efficient production of aggregate-good consequences. In particular, the autonomy of persons (including the autonomy to take health risks) and justice in the distribution of benefits from health programs are crucial moral criteria. Even if nonmorally basic care was cost-effective, it would not follow that it was morally basic in the sense of meeting all moral criteria including the criteria of justice.

Inadequate Attention to Justice

This second problem is perhaps the most serious one raised by the Oregon experiment in its present form. The QWB index used by the Health Services Commission (or any other QALY calculation) is designed to calculate an index of aggregate benefit from the alternative uses of resources.[8] Whether the commission's original cost-benefit formula or only an aggregate net benefits measure is used, in principle the methodology is designed so that the distribution of benefits among recipients cannot have an impact. The adjustments made by the commissioners to the ranking are said to permit adjustment for consideration of equity, but before examining the soundness of that defense, it is necessary to see exactly what is at stake.

What is critical is recognizing that the plan that produces the most net benefit (that is, net benefit per unit of resources once the budget for medicaid is fixed) may not be morally the best plan. The principle of justice requires that social policy consider not only the aggregate amount of benefit but also the morality of the distribution of the benefits. In principle, a QWB index or QALY cannot directly measure the distribution of benefits.*

Several examples of the concern over justice in the Oregon experiment may make the problem clearer. According to the formal principle of justice, equals should be treated equally. The commissioners appear to interpret this to mean that persons in medically similar situations should receive the same treatment. However, establishing priorities raises questions of the material principles of justice.

The problem first appears when one asks why, if people medically similar should be treated equally, the program only covers persons up to 100 percent of the poverty level. Presumably, the answer is that persons above that level, even if they are in a medically similar situation, are nevertheless better off, given their greater economic resources.

Then the question arises of why one would not argue that those far below the poverty line are analogously worse off than those who are less far below it. On some widely accepted theories of justice, material principles of justice require that social practices (such as health insurance programs) be arranged to benefit the least well-off. Although that easily explains why medicaid should focus on those below the poverty level rather than those above it, it equally well explains why the program should give more benefits to those far below poverty than those less far below. From the point of view of justice, it is paradoxical that the Oregon program is going to divert some benefits from the poorest to the somewhat less poor. Justice would seem to suggest just the opposite policy.

My concern is that the Oregon methodology has no mechanism for even considering this kind of claim. It ranks condition-treatment pairs and does not consider whether the benefit of the intervention goes to the very worst off or those who are better off. At the stage at which the computer ranked net benefits, there is no way the data on to whom the benefits accrue could influence the ranking.

---

*Indirectly, these scales would reflect distribution insofar as inequalities of distribution tend to decrease the amount of good. If there is decreasing marginal utility then, as Mill points out, more equal arrangements will produce greater good. The problem in health care, however, is that frequently there is not decreasing marginal utility in health care interventions. The sickest, the worst off, are less efficient to treat, not more efficient. In that case inequalities in the distribution of health resources are cost-effective.

Consider a hypothetical pair of diagnoses, one of which was a problem predominantly afflicting the poorest, while the other was a problem primarily afflicting somewhat better-off patients. The net benefit and cost-benefit formulas used by the commission would be absolutely indifferent between the two problems; in fact, the formulas would not be able to distinguish them. A principle of justice would give a clear priority to a condition that manifests itself primarily among the poorest.

A variant on this problem arises if one considers two condition-treatment pairs each of which would, according to the calculations, produce the same net benefit. Suppose one of the interventions would add a total of one quality-adjusted year to persons with five years to live who were currently living poor-quality lives (say at the 0.3 level). Suppose the second intervention would also add a total of one quality-adjusted life year to persons with five years to live who were currently living relatively high-quality lives (say at the 0.7 level). The formula tells us that the two interventions would produce exactly the same net benefit (one quality-adjusted life year); the commmission's methodology would reveal absolutely no difference between the two. It seems obvious, however, that justice requires giving higher priority to raising people from the 0.3 to the 0.5 level than to raising people from the 0.7 to the 0.9 level.

There is another variant on this justice problem that the commission formulas cannot accommodate. Suppose that how poor one was correlated with one's judgment of how much benefit would be received from a particular intervention. Suppose that data showed that better-off persons considered the net benefit of intervening to treat a sickle cell crisis to be smaller than worse-off persons did. (Given the racial correlates of social class, this hypothesis is not implausible.) Justice would seem to require giving greater weight to the benefit assessment of those who are worse off. In fact, the commissioners, the community meetings, and the Health Care Parliament from which data were gathered disproportionately reflect relatively prosperous persons, not the poorest patients at all.[9] In any case, the commission methodology cannot accommodate such social variations in assessing benefit.

One final example of how justice might be considered comes from the problem of what can be called voluntary health risks.[10] Some health benefits can be offered to people who suffer health detriments through their own voluntary life-style choices. If justice requires that the practice of health insurance be arranged to give people opportunities to be healthy, then it could be argued that a given net benefit from an intervention for conditions beyond people's control has a moral priority over the same amount of benefit for conditions brought on by voluntary health risks. Of course, whether such a policy is adopted will depend not only on the moral judgment about whether justice supports this reasoning but also on whether a particular risk is voluntarily undertaken. The point is that the formulas calculating net benefit and cost-benefit ratios cannot consider this.

There are similar concerns about justice that the formulas cannot account for. Some would argue that justice requires opportunities for well-being over a lifetime, the implication of which is that younger persons would have stronger claims of justice to equal net benefits than older persons—or at least that those who have lived a full, normal life-span have lower priority for certain services.[11] The commission's formula could have taken this partly into account by using the years of expected benefit based on the actual ages of beneficiaries. Instead, it used years of expected benefit of the person at the median age of onset.*

The commission and its defenders have indicated that, although the original cost-benefit ratio formula itself cannot consider the concerns of justice in distribution, the commissioners made several adjustments. First, for the February 1991 rankings, they used the computerized determination of net benefit rather than of the cost-benefit ratio.[12] That would permit a high ranking for a treatment perceived as very beneficial, yet expensive. Insofar as this increases access to the least well-off, it would promote justice. It would not, however, permit any direct consideration of whether benefits accrue to the least advantaged. It would not favor a treatment moving someone from 0.3 to 0.5 on the quality-of-well-being scale over a treatment moving someone from 0.7 to 0.9.

Second, seventeen categories of interventions were ranked based

---

*Even this adjustment would not account for the claim of justice that would give priority to a young person over an older person when the years of life expectancy are the same. Consider, for example, the claim that a twenty-year-old with five years to live has a claim of justice over an eighty-year-old with the same life expectancy because the eighty-year-old has already had sixty extra years. Merely using actual age at onset rather than median age would not account for a sense that younger persons have a priority in justice over older persons with the same life expectancy.

on three attributes, each incorporating several of a total of thirteen health-related values. As far as I can tell, only the attribute, "value to an individual at risk of needing the service," could possibly incorporate concerns for justice. It at least contained "equity" as one of the values.

It is almost impossible, however, to see how the concerns about justice described here could significantly affect the rankings by means of the commissioners' assessment of "value to an individual." In the first place, "equity" is only one of ten values included in the "value to an individual" attribute, which, in turn, is only one of three attributes. Even if some way could have been found by which commissioners could factor in justice, its impact would probably have been minimal.

More critically, justice is not at all about how valuable a service is to a person needing it; it is about the relative claims of different persons needing the services. I do not see how the equity factor in this attribute could, even in theory, permit justice to enter into the ranking of the categories. Even if it did, it would not affect the ranking of the condition-treatment pair except insofar as one whole category generated a justice claim which placed it higher than others. But since the categories are so general, that seems implausible. For all of these reasons, I am forced to conclude that it is simply impossible for the commission to have considered the principle of justice either in the computerized rankings or in the ranking of the categories.

That leaves only one place in which justice could play a role: in the subjective adjustment process that occurred after the categories were ranked and the individual condition-treatment pairs were ranked within categories according to computer-generated net benefit data. Justice may have had some consideration here. For example, liver transplant for alcoholic cirrhosis of the liver was given a final ranking of 690, while transplant for cirrhosis of the liver not involving alcohol was ranked 366, even though the outcome for alcoholic cirrhosis is as good or even better.

It is impossible to determine what role, if any, justice played in the subjective adjustments in the ranking. But that is precisely my point. An incredibly sophisticated method was developed and tested at enormous expense to have a computer generate net benefit and cost-benefit data for each of the hundreds of condition-treatment pairs. Nothing comparable was developed to account for the justice of the rankings.

Such methods could have been tried. For example, by using the data already in the computer measuring how poorly off persons were, the commission could have written algorithms to consider in ranking whether the benefits accrue to very sick persons or to healthier persons. By adding data on the relation between income level and incidence rates, the commission could have written algorithms considering how poorly off economically the patients were. The computer could have been programmed to make use of the data indicating how well off persons were in absolute terms as well as how much net benefit was produced. A standardized index of how poorly off the beneficiaries were (in medical or economic terms, or both) could have been calculated. Then the commission could have made a conscious policy decision establishing the relative importance of the net benefit of an intervention to the justness of the intervention.

For example, the United Network for Organ Sharing Ethics Committee Allocation Subcommittee has adopted the position that medical benefit and justice should be considered equally important in allocation decisions. In the Oregon Plan virtually the entire ranking is driven by estimates of net benefit, with only vague, subjective, afterthought adjustments considering justice. Moreover, because it is condition-treatment pairs that are ranked, there is, in principle, no way to distinguish within a specific intervention between more- and less-just claims to a particular pair.

Inability to Differentiate within a Condition-Treatment Pair

This raises a final serious problem with the Oregon experiment as it is evolving. The product of the commission's work will be a ranking of condition-treatment pairs that allows the legislature to draw a line by appropriating a specific budget that, based on actuarial calculations, will fund down the list to a cutoff point. This means that the entire process precludes any differentiation of more- and less-weighty claims within a particular condition-treatment. As discussed, different people would not be able to have different claims of justice to a particular condition-treatment according to how well or poorly off they were, economically and medically.

For example, neuroplasty for peripheral nerve injury ranks 36 even though some such injuries must be much more serious than others. It seems impossible for the *system* to distinguish between injuries so minor that surgery might well be forgone and those so severe that major hardship would be suffered without the surgery.

Even more important, there seems no way to differentiate among marginal and more critical aspects of a treatment. Consider, for example, appendectomy for appendicitis. It will come as no surprise that it ranks fifth on the list of 709 interventions. It takes no great talent to realize that appendectomy is worth funding, at least for clear-cut diagnosis of appendicitis.

The real issue is not whether to perform the appendectomy; it is whether to fund countless marginal interventions that are potentially part of the procedure—marginal blood tests and repeat tests; precautionary, preventive antibiotic therapy before surgery; the number of nurses in the operating room; and the backup support on call or in the hospital. Even more decisions about marginal elements will arise during the recovery phase—exactly how many days of hospital stay are permitted, how often the physician should make rounds, how many follow-up tests there should be, and so on. Many of these are predicted to offer more benefits than harm, but with margins so small that one could argue that resources ought to be used elsewhere. Clearly, every last element of intervention should not be provided to the point at which the intervention is predicted to do as much harm as good; that would be irresponsibly inefficient.

The Oregon ranking ignores the possibility of increasing efficiency and fairness in the medicaid program by racheting down on the inefficient and unfair elements within any given treatment and of eliminating cases of marginal need for a high-priority service. Surely, marginal instances of a particular diagnosis have less of a claim than full-fledged ones, and marginal elements of a treatment are less important than the critical elements. Eliminating marginal elements of a treatment is probably more important in creating an ethically responsible allocation than deciding exactly what the priority ranking is among the 709 diagnoses. Certainly, the criteria of medical benefit and justice require that the system be able to make such judgments in a systematic and fair way.

CONCLUSION

These three problems—the equivocation between uses of the term *basic* in its moral and nonmoral senses, the inadequate attention to justice, and the inability to differentiate within condition-treatment pairs—are serious problems that must be addressed if the important experiment in Oregon is to be successful. In the end, rationing is both inevitable and morally necessary. The key is that it be done with an explicit sense of the moral principles underlying it. If those doing the rationing assume, without examination, that the morally correct allocation is the one that produces the most efficient aggregate good and further assume that care that is low-tech, preventive, or primary is necessarily the most efficient at producing benefits, serious errors will be made. If these questions are explored thoroughly before the key rationing decisions are made, resource allocation will serve the community effectively.

NOTES

1. The argument for the inevitability and moral necessity of rationing is developed fully in Robert M. Veatch, "Physicians and Cost Containment: The Ethical Conflict," *Jurimetrics Journal*, vol. 30 (Summer 1990), pp. 461–82.

2. Robert M. Kaplan, "Quality of Life Measurement," in Paul Karoly, ed., *Measurement Strategies in Health Psychology* (New York: Wiley-Interscience, 1985), pp. 5–46.

3. Milton C. Weinstein and William B. Stason, "Foundations of Cost-Effectiveness Analysis for Health and Medical Practices," *New England Journal of Medicine*, vol. 296 (March 31, 1977), pp. 716–21.

4. Norman Daniels, "Is the Oregon Rationing Plan Fair?" *Journal of the American Medical Association*, vol. 265 (May 1, 1991), pp. 2232–35.

5. Dan E. Beauchamp and Ronald L. Rouse, "Universal New York Health Care: A Single-Payor Strategy Linking Cost Control and Universal Access," *New England Journal of Medicine*, vol. 323 (September 6, 1990), pp. 640–44.

6. Oregon Health Services Commission, *Prioritization of Health Services* (1991), p. G-9.

7. John Kitzhaber, "A Healthier Approach to Health Care," *Issues in Science and Technology*, vol. 7 (Winter 1990–91), pp. 59–65.

8. Oregon Health Services Commission, *Prioritization of Health Services*, p. D-2.

9. Ralph Crawshaw and others, "Developing Principles for Prudent Health Care Allocation: The Continuing Oregon Experiment," *Western Journal of Medicine*, vol. 152 (April 1990), pp. 441–46.

10. Robert M. Veatch, "Voluntary Risks to Health: The Ethical Issues," *Journal of the American Medical Association*, vol. 243 (January 4, 1980), pp. 50–55.

11. Robert M. Veatch, "Distributive Justice and the Allocation of Technolog-

ical Resources to the Elderly," in *Life-Sustaining Technologies and the Elderly: Working Papers,* vol. 3: *Legal and Ethical Issues, Manpower and Training, and Classification Systems for Decisionmaking* (Washington: Office of Technology Assessment, 1987), pp. 87–189; Norman Daniels, *Am I My Parents' Keeper? An Essay on Justice between the Young and the Old* (Oxford University Press, 1988); and Daniel Callahan, *Setting Limits: Medical Goals in an Aging Society* (Simon and Schuster, 1987).

12. Oregon Health Services Commission, *Prioritization of Health Services,* p. G-15.

S A R A   R O S E N B A U M

Poor Women, Poor Children, Poor Policy: The Oregon Medicaid Experiment

My analysis of Oregon's proposed public and private health insurance reform package focuses on one aspect of the state's proposal—its plan to reduce medicaid benefits for approximately 100,000 current beneficiaries, virtually all of whom are the state's poorest women of child-bearing age and their children. The proposal to reduce medicaid benefits for currently eligible women and children is part of a larger set of legislative changes aimed at increasing health insurance coverage for many of the state's uninsured residents. It is the medicaid reduction component of the state's proposal, however, that lies at the heart of the controversy. Those aspects of the package that would extend medicaid to currently ineligible persons, mandate minimum health benefits for many workers and their families, and establish public insurance mechanisms for the medically uninsurable are all worthwhile. Indeed, many states are now pursuing, or have enacted, similar proposals even in these difficult fiscal times.

BACKGROUND

It is important to begin by reviewing the basic aspects of the state's medicaid reduction plan. Essentially, the state seeks permission—either administratively, through federal research and demonstration authority granted by the secretary of the Department of Health and Human Services (HHS) under section 1115 of the Social Security Act, or legislatively, by act of Congress, or both—to receive substantial additional federal medicaid payments to cover certain uninsured poor

I gratefully acknowledge Larissa Jones, of the Georgetown University Law Center, for her assistance on the section that pertains to federally conducted biomedical and behavioral research involving human subjects.

persons while at the same time diverging from current law in two important respects. First, the state would eliminate coverage of medically necessary federally mandated benefits from its medicaid plan for certain beneficiaries. Coverage would be denied if a patient's condition or diagnosis and the type of treatment prescribed were to fall below a specified cutoff point on a "prioritized" list of condition-treatment pairs. Current federal medicaid regulations prohibit arbitrary limitations on required services based on a patient's condition or diagnosis.[1] The condition-treatment pairs that fall below the initial cutoff point proposed by the state include some that have been classified by the Oregon Health Services Commission as either "essential," "very important," or "valuable."[2]

Second, the state seeks waivers that would allow it to obtain federal funding to help offset the cost of extending medicaid to persons whose eligibility for coverage is not now recognized under federal law. These persons include a small number of poor children.[3] Most of the new beneficiaries, however, are single adults and childless couples who are neither disabled nor elderly and who therefore are categorically ineligible for coverage under current law.

The state does not allege that the omitted condition-treatment pairs are medically unnecessary (for which no federal medicaid funding can be claimed under current law even in the absence of waivers).[4] Nor does the state claim that the treatments to be denied are either medically ineffective or experimental. The omitted treatments are those "very important" or "effective" treatments that the commission has ranked excessively costly, given the quality of life that can be expected in light of both the patient's underlying condition or diagnosis and the public and social value attached to the treatment for that condition.

Oregon clearly has the latitude to use, without prior federal approval, a condition-treatment prioritization mechanism in programs that are entirely state funded and that are not subject to federal requirements. For example, the state could establish a public health insurance plan funded by state and local revenues for all its uninsured residents, and it could use prioritization to allocate resources. No federal authorization would be needed. The state could require all employers either to provide benefits that meet the mandates of this hypothetical state plan or to contribute to the cost of the plan. Similarly, the state could incorporate a condition-treatment prioritization mechanism into its own state employee benefit plan without federal waivers. In short, the state could test this system tomorrow—free of either federal funding or congressional oversight.

What brings the state to Washington, D.C., is its desire to obtain sizable federal medicaid funds to help underwrite the cost of its plan. It is this request for hundreds of millions of dollars in federal revenues that demands particularly close scrutiny. This is particularly true of the aspect of the plan that affects current medicaid beneficiaries by withdrawing medically necessary care for the approximately 75 percent of the state's current medicaid population who are women of childbearing age and children. These beneficiaries would not be provided with a fixed benefit package. Instead, they would be covered by a plan whose diagnostically driven coverage rules would be permitted to constrict even more if actual costs exceed the state's budget projections.

The state does not claim (although initially it did) that its prioritization system would allow it to cover both current and new beneficiaries for the same amount now spent on medicaid for the experimental population of current beneficiaries. Indeed, recent actuarial estimates indicate that the proposal would cost both the state and federal governments tens of millions of dollars in additional funding annually. Given the federal medicaid financial contribution level to which the state is entitled, the demonstration authority Oregon seeks would provide it with much greater federal assistance.

The additional federal funding required to implement the state's medicaid plan would warrant careful examination even under normal conditions. These are not normal times. Under the terms of the Budget Act Amendments of 1990, any additional funding needed to implement the Oregon Plan (assuming that its implementation is determined by the secretary of HHS not to be budget neutral) will necessitate either the imposition of new taxes or specific cuts in other federal entitlement programs, such as medicare, social security and aid to families with dependent children (AFDC). A threshold question, therefore, is whether, as a matter of public policy, the state should receive such large sums at a time when many federal programs for the poor are in great need of expansion nationwide.[5]

This is especially true because the plan has been characterized by the state as particularly helpful to women and children. Yet, it is now competing for funding against other congressional medicaid proposals to aid poor women and children in all states. Current proposals include legislation to extend medicaid to all pregnant women and infants with family incomes below 185 percent of the federal poverty level, provide states the option of covering all children with family incomes below 185 percent of the federal poverty level, improve the scope of care for poor pregnant women and infants, strengthen state medicaid immunization programs, and improve medicaid coverage for migrant children and women of childbearing age.

Given the urgency of all these measures and the significant spending constraints under which Congress and the president have elected to place themselves as a result of the 1990 budget agreement, the Oregon Plan should be funded only if its value to children is perceived as unmatched. Its adoption would consume a large proportion of the limited federal funding that might otherwise be available to advance one or more of these competing national initiatives.

The Oregon Plan would affect only a single state. By contrast, the competing proposals would, in at least one case, relieve states entirely of the financial burden of covering low-income pregnant women and infants. (Pending legislation mandating coverage of all pregnant women and infants with family incomes below 185 percent of the federal poverty level would be accompanied by fully federalized medicaid payments.) The other proposals would provide states with valuable federal funding to help all poor children.

If a decision is made that the Oregon Plan potentially merits more investment than other national medicaid proposals, the next question is whether the plan, as crafted, is a meritorious experiment. If, as noted, the Oregon Plan were authorized administratively by the secretary, permission would come under the legislative power delegated to the secretary under section 1115 of the Social Security Act.[6] If Congress itself were to grant the state's request legislatively, it presumably would do so because it considered the state's proposal a valuable piece of health services research, not merely a new way to reduce medicaid benefits to poor people. Therefore, assuming that the cost of the demonstration is not intrinsically a fundamental barrier to legislative or administrative action at this point, two crucial questions must precede any decision to grant or to deny the state's request. Can a proposal that eliminates coverage of medically necessary care for poor medicaid-enrolled children and women of childbearing age be considered the type of legitimate federal research that the secretary is authorized to pursue under section 1115 of the Social Security Act? And if the answer to this question is yes, then must research safeguards be included, and what should these safeguards consist of?

OBJECTIONS TO THE OREGON PLAN

In my opinion, given the current scope and structure of the medicaid program for children, Oregon's proposal does not further any legitimate objectives of the Social Security Act and thus falls outside the scope of the secretary's section 1115 powers. The plan should not be funded if it eliminates medically necessary care for currently enrolled poor children. Moreover, if an administrative or legislative decision is made to authorize the proposal, the plan clearly constitutes research involving human subjects. Federal regulations governing such research compel the inclusion of certain fundamental safeguards.

The Problem of Legitimate Research

The proposal does not represent the type of research that furthers the objectives of the medicaid program, given current medicaid standards governing eligibility and benefits for children.

For administrative waivers to be granted by the secretary under the Social Security Act's section 1115 demonstration provision, the proposed research must be of a type consistent with the objectives of the particular Social Security Act program under whose auspices the demonstration is to occur. If a decision is made to conduct this demonstration through a grant of legislative authority, then it should be assumed that Congress, in granting such authority, will wish to promote the objectives of the medicaid statute. The starting point, therefore, is an assessment of the objectives of the medicaid statute. In particular, an assessment must be made of the act's objectives for children, because, in the case of Oregon's experiment, two-thirds of the experimental current beneficiary group are children.

In recent years federal medicaid standards for children have been sweepingly altered. To be consistent with medicaid's objectives for children, the demonstration should be consistent with these reforms. The Oregon proposal, far from being consistent with recent reforms, establishes a precedent for gutting them.

Since virtually the inception of the program, medicaid benefits for children have been governed by special, generous federal protections. Children constitute nearly half of all medicaid recipients nationally, and because of medicaid's tie to the eroding AFDC program, children historically have been the poorest of all recipients.[7]

The special standards guaranteeing enriched medicaid benefits for children are both warranted and increasingly urgent. Childhood poverty is significantly greater today than it was a generation ago,[8] and private health insurance coverage for children has eroded markedly.[9] In many states, high rates of childhood poverty and disinsurance rates have combined to make medicaid a primary source of maternity and pediatric health care financing.[10] Therefore, any proposal that would eliminate some "very important" and "valuable" services for children should be viewed with special concern.

Actions by Congress in recent years reflect strong recognition of the special role played by medicaid in maternal and child health. In recent years, Congress has amended federal law to require coverage of children under age six and all pregnant women with family income below 133 percent of the federal poverty level and all children ages six to nineteen with family incomes under 100 percent of poverty.[11]

Congress also expanded medicaid to provide additional health benefits to enrolled children. For nearly twenty-five years, federal law has required states to provide to all children eligible for medicaid a special package of benefits known collectively as early and periodic screening, diagnosis, and treatment (EPSDT).[12] Added to medicaid in 1967, in response to overwhelming evidence regarding the diminished health status of poor children and youth, EPSDT is designed to ensure comprehensive health coverage and the prevention of long-term health problems. It provides to all medicaid-enrolled children under twenty-one expanded benefits for a broad range of primary and preventive treatment. It also guarantees treatment for physical, mental, and developmental conditions and disabilities disclosed during a child's health exam (known as a screen).

In 1989, responding to evidence of serious shortcomings in the program, Congress revised and extended EPSDT in a number of ways.[13] Two of the revisions are directly relevant to this discussion. The first amendment revoked states' authority to apply benefit limitations in their EPSDT programs that excluded any diagnostic and treatment services for which federal medicaid payments could be claimed.[14] Essentially, the amendment mandated for children the provision of all services otherwise classified in the statute as optional in the case of adults. As a result of the 1989 amendments, for example, a state no longer has the right to elect to exclude coverage of physical therapy (otherwise an optional service for adults) from its state plan in the case of children. If a child's screening exam reveals a need for physical therapy, coverage must be provided even if it is not a covered benefit under the state's plan for persons over age twenty-one.

The second relevant 1989 EPSDT amendment provided that, in setting limitations (known in medicaid parlance as "amount, duration, and scope" limitations) for covered benefits, states must, for children, use only limitations that are consistent with the preventive purposes of EPSDT and must cover all medically necessary care.[15] For example, if a child's exam shows a need for hospital and physician care, the state may deny payment only if the care and services are not medically necessary to achieve the preventive purposes of the EPSDT program. This standard applies even if the medically necessary care and services needed to prevent long-term health problems could be denied adults. Thus, although a state might permissibly limit hospital coverage to only eighteen days a year for adults, regardless of a particular condition or their need for care (indeed, this is a limitation that Oregon currently employs), for children, the 1989 federal medical necessity standard would compel coverage of all medically necessary care.

Taken together, the two EPSDT amendments mandate coverage of virtually all services for which federal reimbursement can be claimed, and outlaw the use of coverage limitations based on considerations other than whether a service is medically necessary to achieve the program's preventive purpose. Therefore, research conducted pursuant to section 1115 of the Social Security Act that has either the intent or the effect of withdrawing coverage for medically necessary care on the basis of a poor child's condition is not consistent with the objectives of the statute, and waivers should not be granted.*

In the case of adults, the argument might be made that the prioriti-

---

*The state's proposal also appears to eliminate medicaid coverage for many of the poor children recently added to the program, by using a more stringent test of poverty than the one used in the statute. This proposal alone renders the plan inconsistent with the objectives for the Social Security Act.

zation approach is no more harmful than existing law, since the statute now gives states latitude to cut back on or deny benefits. But this argument is flawed even for adults because the current medicaid program, despite its weaknesses, at least guarantees adults a minimum benefit package and prohibits discrimination against adults with disabilities. The argument is utterly without merit as regards children, however. Recognizing their extreme poverty, their vulnerable health status, the value of comprehensive care, and their extraordinary dependence on medicaid, Congress has underscored its intent that medicaid play a particularly expansive role for children—a role that goes well beyond that which it plays for adults. To sanction an experiment that effectively unravels all that Congress has done to improve medicaid for children goes against the statute.

If Oregon elects to use its own funds to insure children who are ineligible for medicaid for less than all medically necessary care, it obviously has the right to do so. Certainly, for such children, some coverage undoubtedly would be better than none. But where federal funding is concerned, Congress has decreed that all poor children be covered and that all covered children be provided with all medically necessary care. For the secretary of HHS to abrogate that coverage under his federal demonstration authority would amount to sanctioning research that is not consistent with medicaid's objectives for children, and conceivably could be considered an abuse of agency discretion. Were Congress to authorize the experiment, it would effectively repeal its own medicaid child health amendments and go against nearly a decade of incremental efforts to improve and strengthen the way medicaid helps children.

The Problem of Safeguards

If the state does receive approval to proceed with its plan to reduce children's benefits, then certain research safeguards must be adhered to.

Assuming that a decision is made to proceed with the state's proposal and grant its request for federal waivers and additional federal funds, then it is essential that such research be conducted only in conformity with the protections and safeguards that apply to federally funded biomedical and behavioral research involving human subjects. These protections are compelled by the very nature of the Oregon experiment, which would deny essential medical care to the poorest people. They also are warranted because of Congress's longstanding concern with federally conducted research involving human subjects. Furthermore, considering that the human subjects involved in this federally financed experiment are overwhelmingly women of childbearing age and children, the level of research protection accorded the experimental population should be comprehensive.

Regulations governing HHS-provided biomedical and behavioral research involving humans impose stringent requirements.[16] The rules are designed to ensure that the level of risk involved does not outweigh the benefits to be gained from the research, and, if allowed to proceed, that the research is accompanied by certain safeguards. Federally funded research under medicaid, such as that proposed by Oregon, which tests the impact of withdrawing coverage for medically necessary care, has been recognized as research properly within the scope of human subject protections by the Department of Health and Human Services, federal courts, and congressionally created bodies established to advise the secretary of HHS on protections involving human subjects.[17]

The proposal before the HHS and Congress constitutes biomedical research by definition. It would withdraw coverage from an exceedingly poor population for some health services that, by the applicant's own admission, are "very important" and "valuable." Moreover, *the experiment explicitly sanctions the withdrawal of health care by providers treating experimental populations*. It does so by modifying common law tort principles to eliminate the legal liability that providers otherwise would face were they to abandon patients who needed medical care but who had lost their health insurance.[18] As a result, at stake is not only the financial underwriting of health insurance for poor people but also their access to the very services themselves.

Since the 1960s the HHS has regulated biomedical and behavioral research involving human subjects. Regulations promulgated in 1981 pursuant to the National Research Act and the secretary's general rulemaking authority extend basic research protections to all biomedical and behavioral research conducted by, or funded in whole or in part by, the department.[19] This research includes federally funded research conducted pursuant to the secretary's Social Security Act research authority.

Central to the protection of human subjects is review of proposed experiments by an independent institutional review board (IRB)—or, in the case of section 1115 projects, by department officials—to determine whether the benefits of the experiment to those affected outweigh its risks.[20] Only in the event that federally funded biomedical research involving humans meets this threshold test can the experiment proceed, and then only with certain safeguards such as voluntary participation, informed consent, and special protections should the experimental group consist of children or other vulnerable populations.[21]

In comments to the Department of Health and Human Services in 1982, following a proposal by the Reagan administration to entirely exempt research conducted under Social Security Act programs from human subject protections,[22] the President's Commission for the Study of Ethics in Medicine and Biomedical and Behavioral Research argued that impartial scientific review by an independent IRB was a fundamental protection for all federally supported research involving human subjects. The commission proposed the following standard for determining when no IRB review of human subject research conducted under section 1115 of the Social Security Act would be needed:

> These regulations do not apply to research designed to evaluate federally sponsored social, economic or health programs where (1) the appropriate departmental official has been given explicit Congressional authority to modify a program for research purposes, (2) the programs or changes are themselves within the statutory authority of the agency to adopt, *and* (3) the research involves no limitation or withholding of a benefit to which the subjects are legally entitled or which other individuals, similarly situated, continue to receive under the current program being evaluated [emphasis added].[23]

The case for human subject review is particularly compelling in the Oregon context. The crux of the research is the withdrawal of medically necessary care from indigent persons otherwise entitled to medicaid coverage for the care and services to be denied. This is research involving human subjects at its most profound. Moreover, only the most politically vulnerable medicaid recipients, two-thirds of whom are children, are to be subjected to the experiment—at least initially. This raises the degree of concern to an even higher level, because traditionally research involving children has been permitted to proceed only with the utmost safeguards.

In recent legislation involving federally financed research on medicaid beneficiaries, Congress has chosen to adhere to the principle of protection articulated by the commission. In 1982, after promulgation of an "emergency" rule by the Reagan administration bypassing human subject protections in federally conducted medicaid copayment experiments,[24] Congress added to the medicaid statute itself a provision requiring certain basic safeguards for medicaid beneficiary cost-sharing experiments.[25] These safeguards include both an IRB-level review by HHS and additional safeguards for members of the experimental group. The congressional protections articulated for copayment experiments should be viewed as a base on which protections for beneficiaries of the Oregon experiment (if allowed to proceed) are to be built, because copayment experiments entail a far less significant reduction in benefits than those that will be imposed under the Oregon Plan.

I now turn to the minimum protections that should accompany the granting of a waiver to Oregon. First, and perhaps most fundamental, the proposal should, like all biomedical and behavioral research involving human subjects, be reviewed by an independent IRB. An IRB, unlike current administration officials (who by their own admission have worked in close collaboration with the state to design the waiver), is in a position to make an impartial judgment about whether the benefits to the experimental population of this piece of research outweigh its risks. An independent IRB review would correctly focus on the research subjects themselves—that is, current medicaid beneficiary children—rather than on persons who might potentially benefit (those currently uninsured) as the experiment unfolds.

Much has been said about the potential benefits of this research to the currently uninsured. But ethics and law demand that the research also be of value to the persons whose benefits will be withdrawn. Speculation about potential value cannot conceal the fact that if this research proceeds, tens of thousands of currently insured poor children will lose coverage for medically necessary health services and will have their legal claims for care extinguished under common law tort principles. Because of longstanding ethical principles, this federally sanctioned withdrawal of life-and-death benefits from a highly politically vulnerable population cannot be allowed to proceed without independent IRB review.

If the proposal survives a threshold IRB risk-benefit review, further protections should be added. First, the medicaid portion of the plan should be allowed to proceed only when Oregon's companion bill mandating private coverage in accordance with the prioritized-care list goes into effect for all currently uninsured Oregonians—not only those who will be covered through a restructured medicaid plan. It is my understanding that the effective date of the employer mandate portion of the state's package is 1995. This date should govern the medicaid waiver date as well. Such a direct linkage would mitigate, though by no means remove, the problems caused by subjecting only the poorest state residents not only to the initial experiment but also to the possibility of further deep cuts during the experimental period should funds fall short of what is needed to finance the system at its initial cutoff.[26]

The IRB should also develop special safeguards for the experimental population. These safeguards might mirror those now contained in the medicaid statute that governs cost-sharing experiments. These safeguards require either that participation be voluntary or that a state arrange to compensate persons suffering injury or death as a result of the experimental withholding of medically necessary care involuntarily. Alternatively, the IRB might fashion a different approach, such as requiring supplemental state and federal funding to cover the cost of medically necessary care disallowed under the experimental plan. Under this arrangement, current beneficiaries denied otherwise covered care would nonetheless receive it. They could then be followed for several years to determine the ultimate effectiveness of the care that would have been denied in the absence of this research "safety net."

Both safeguards would be justified in this case. Assumption of legal liability by the state for injuries caused helps offset the fact that the Oregon Plan would, as noted, modify common law tort principles and insulate medicaid providers from civil or criminal liability or disciplinary sanctions for failing to treat beneficiaries for conditions whose treatment is excluded from the plan.[27] The second proposal— to pay for care that otherwise would be disallowed and then to follow the resulting care patterns—can be justified in light of the admittedly shaky factual basis for the prioritization system itself.[28]

CONCLUSION

There is no question that the plight of America's 35 to 37 million un-insured persons, at least one-quarter of whom are children, compels action. Limitations on tax-supported health expenditures for all Americans would be one way to provide the financial resources necessary to insure these individuals. This choice is one that many countries have made as part of an overall national health plan that allocates available health resources for an entire population.

Oregon, however, does not seek the federal authority to reallocate overall state health resources in a more equitable fashion. Indeed, the state does not even propose to subject its own state-financed state employee health benefit plan to the prioritization system. Instead, "prioritization" is reserved for the weakest and poorest state residents—women and children living at less than half the federal poverty level and utterly dependent on direct state assistance.

Thus far, the state's response to the concerns that the Children's Defense Fund and many others have raised has been basically two-fold. First, the state argues, rationing must begin somewhere, and the plan would have failed had it begun with the more politically powerful. Second, the state insists, the political process itself will protect the subjects of this experiment, because public opinion will not allow the experimental group's coverage to sink below acceptable levels.

The fundamental inconsistency between these two statements is striking. Why should anyone believe that the very process that pushed 100,000 indigent babies, children, and women into a health care reduction plan will now rise to their rescue as budget shortfalls set in and allocated funding begins to run out? Why should anyone imagine that a state, whose per capita medicaid expenditures on children's behalf has ranked among the lowest in the nation, will rush in with supplemental resources for poor children, particularly after the enormous costs involved in covering nearly 100,000 additional poor adults not previously eligible for medicaid begin to mount up?

The Oregon Plan is not an experiment that can be justified legally, scientifically, programmatically, or ethically. Its proponents argue that it represents the best in hard, tough thinking about the shape of the future health system. In reality, it represents no hard thinking at all. When the smoke clears, the Oregon medicaid reduction plan is only one more in a long series of proposals to reduce benefits to the very poor—a novel one, to be sure, and one that has garnered much attention. But underneath the weighty hypotheses and intricate equations is a medicaid cutback. Only the packaging has changed.

NOTES

1. 42 CFR sec. 440.230 (1991). Since only arbitrary limitations are prohibited, the question arises whether a state's limitations are, in fact, arbitrary, or whether they are based on reasonable medical evidence. If the latter is true, diagnostic exclusions may be permissible under existing law, at least in some instances.

2. Office of the Governor, State of Oregon, "Governor Accepts Final Health Care Priority List, Moves Legislature Toward Fund," May 1, 1991, pp. 1–2.

3. Effective July 1, 1991, all states must extend medicaid coverage on a year-by-year, phased-in basis to all children born after September 1983 who have attained age six but who have not attained age nineteen, and who have family incomes below 100 percent of the federal poverty level. Sec. 4601, P.L. 101-508. Under current law, states must extend coverage to all poor pregnant women, infants, and, therefore, children born after September 30, 1983. 42 USC sec. 1396(a)(10)(A)(i) (1991). Thus, Oregon's medicaid plan has virtually no effect whatsoever on expanding the coverage of poor pregnant women, infants, and young children. Indeed, the state seeks waivers of certain adjustments to income normally available to poor families and children applying for benefits. If these waivers are granted, potentially thousands of otherwise eligible poor children with gross incomes above the federal poverty level, but net incomes below it, will be denied coverage.

4. 42 USC sec. 1396a(a)(30)(A) (1991).

5. It is worth noting that fifteen years ago Oregon also received millions of dollars in additional federal medicaid funding to extend coverage to all poor residents of Multnomah County (Portland). This new plan would be the state's second federally funded indigent health care experiment in less than two decades.

6. 42 USC sec. 1315.

7. Between 1970 and 1990 real-dollar AFDC benefit levels fell by about 40 percent. Children's Defense Fund, *The State of America's Children* (Washington, 1991).

8. Children's Defense Fund, "Children in Poverty," Washington, June 1991.

9. U.S. Bipartisan Commission on Health Care, *A Call to Action* (Washington, 1990).

10. For example, unpublished state data on the proportion of births fi-

nanced by medicaid, reported to the Children's Defense Fund (Summer 1991), show the proportion of all births financed by medicaid to be between 30 and 40 percent in twenty reporting states.

11. 42 USC sec. 1396(a)(10)(A)(i)(VI) and (VII) as added by sec. 6401, P.L. 101-239, and sec. 4402, P.L. 101-508.

12. 42 USC secs. 1396a(a)(10)(A)(i) and 1396d(a)(4)(B) (1991).

13. Sec. 6403, P.L. 101-239 (1989).

14. 42 USC sec. 1396d(r)(5) (1991).

15. Ibid.

16. 45 CFR sec. 46 (1990).

17. See, for example, 45 CFR sec. 4601; *Crane* v. *Mathews*, 417 F. Supp. 532 (ED GA, 1976); and President's Commission for the Study of Ethics in Medicare and Biomedical and Behavioral Research, *Implementing Human Research Regulations: Second Biennial Report on the Adequacy and Uniformity of Federal Rules and Policies and of Their Implementation for the Protection of Human Subjects* (March 1983), pp. 176–80.

18. O.R.S. 414.745 (1990).

19. 46 Reg. 12276 (January 26, 1981).

20. 45 CFR sec. 101. In 1983 the Reagan administration modified the 1981 regulations to limit application of the protections in the case of research conducted pursuant to section 1115 of the Social Security Act. The modifications eliminated the use of independent institutional review boards to conduct safety reviews. 48 Fed. Reg. 9664 (March 8, 1983). However, the HHS preserved an IRB-level standard of review in its internal evaluation of section 1115 biomedical research. It also preserved such basic safeguards as voluntary informed consent. 48 Fed. Reg. 9667.

21. 45 CFR sec. 46.111.

22. 47 Fed. Reg. 12276 (March 22, 1982).

23. Letter from Morris Abram, chairman, President's Commission, to William Dommel, HHS Office for Protection of Human Subjects, August 4, 1982. Final regulations issued on March 4, 1983 (48 Fed. Reg. 9266), did exempt social security demonstrations from an independent institutional review board. However, the rule provides for internal review to determine if the experiment poses a danger—and the use of informed consent if a danger is found to exist.

24. 47 Fed. Reg. 9208 (March 4, 1982).

25. 42 USC sec. 13960(f), added by sec. 131(b), P.L. 97-248.

26. Sec. 8 of S.B. 44, ordered by the Oregon Senate on April 2, 1991, and amending S.B. 27 (which established the medicaid prioritization program) provides in pertinent part that

(1) If insufficient funds are available during a contract period:
(a) the population of eligible persons determined by law shall not be reduced;

(b) the reimbursement rate for providers and plans established under the contractual agreement shall not be reduced.

(2) In the circumstances described in subsection, (1) of this section, reimbursement shall be adjusted by reducing the health services for the eligible population by eliminating services in the order of priority by the Health Services Commission, starting with the least important and progressing toward the most important.

27. O.R.S. 414.745 (1990).

28. In a chapter perhaps aptly entitled "Methodology: A Combination of Values and Data," the Oregon Health Services Commission lists in its 1991 *Report to the Governor and Legislature* the following steps that were developed to prioritize services in light of the "lack of conclusive studies of effectiveness" (p. 10):

Step 1—Creation of ranking of health service categories and classifications of services.

Step 2—Generation of net benefit used to rank condition-treatment pairs within health services categories.

Step 3—*Commission judgment used in creating the methodology and making adjustments to the prioritized list of health services.* [P. 13, emphasis added.]

The Oregon Experiment

Eight years ago, when William Schwartz, of Tufts New England Medical Center, and I wrote *The Painful Prescription: Rationing Hospital Care* (Brookings, 1984), we were, I believe, somewhat ahead of our time. A number of reviewers reacted to our use of the word *rationing* in connection with health care as though we had shouted an obscenity in church.

Fashions change, however, and it is gratifying to see a growing recognition in the United States that sustained long-term reductions in the growth of health care spending will occur only if we are willing to ration. Let me be clear about what is meant when I use the word *rationing*. I use it to mean the denial to people who have the means to pay for health care some services that promise medical benefits. By that definition, the denial of care to those who are uninsured is not what I call rationing.

This does not imply that I defer in any way to the expressions of indignation about the continuation of that situation in the United States. It is deplorable. It should not be allowed to continue. And, what is not so widely known or pointed out, it would be relatively inexpensive to provide, to the roughly 15 percent of Americans who are currently uninsured, care at the average level available to most people who are insured. In fact, the additional cost for insuring all of those who now lack insurance coverage would total approximately 6 percent of current total health care spending. In an effort to place that figure in context, that is roughly the amount by which health care spending in the United States increases in an average year. Therefore, for that relatively modest cost in additional resources, this shameful blot could be eliminated from the current situation in health care spending.

I also do not use the term *rationing* to refer to the elimination of care that provides no benefits at all—such as the needless torment that we impose on some of the terminally ill in the name of life-extending therapy or the fourth blood chemistry workup that some physicians request in the same day for a given patient. Nor do I use *rationing* to mean the elimination of inefficient methods of providing beneficial care.

In the United States a menu of one-time savings is still available that would save significant amounts of money. These one-time savings include eliminating ineffective therapies, reducing administrative costs, improving efficiency in the production of beneficial care, some cutting, perhaps, of physician salaries and fees, and eliminating unnecessary or unoccupied beds and unused equipment. I do not believe, when we got all through with it, malpractice reform would save us much money, but it certainly would improve the way we use available resources.

None of these needless outlays, however, accounts for an appreciable part of the increase in medical expenses in the United States. The driving force was, is, and will be rapid technological advance. The speed of technological improvement shows every sign of accelerating, with such advances as artificial skin for burn victims and implants for the hearing impaired, which are already available; left-ventricle-assist devices for those who suffer cardiac failure, which are close to being available; a virtual avalanche of potential therapies from recombinant DNA research; and the fruits of new findings in molecular biology.

The pressure on costs is not going to relent. In fact, it is important that outlays continue to grow in the United States because the potential benefits for many patients from these new technologies are going to be enormous.

But the current system also encourages—and this is what we have been hearing about—every sick patient who is insured to demand any service, however small the benefit and however great the cost. The crucial question raised by the issue of rationing is whether we will curtail any of the beneficial care for those with the means to pay. In short, when we talk about rationing, the problem is not that we shamefully allow many Americans to have inadequate financial access to health care. The problem, as Pogo said, is us. It is the fact that when we or any of our family members are ill, and we are insured, we want everything that helps.

If we ration, we want to ensure that curtailing the availability of beneficial care is done fairly and efficiently. We should first eliminate the care with the lowest ratio of benefits to costs. As Jean Thorne observes, in discussing benefits we are not talking about the mechanical output of a computer; we are talking about something that is filtered through social, personal, and ethical evaluations based on informed knowledge about medical outcomes.

From this general discussion of rationing I turn to the specifics of the Oregon Plan, which has three components. Two of the components of the plan are logically distinct from the third, and each should be considered separately. Here I address the component that ranks various medical therapies.

Oregon proposes to address the issue of rationing in the right general way. Unfortunately, I do not think that what the state proposes to do is good enough. There is a grave risk that if the Oregon Plan does badly, it will give a very good idea a bad name.

To be specific, there are three main issues. The first, which I do not think is the most important, elicits a great deal of emotion. Oregon currently ranks thirty-fifth in the nation in per capita acute care medicaid outlays. What the state proposes to do can be characterized as funding part of the cost of extending coverage for those who are not now covered in Oregon by cutting benefits for those who are covered. That is undoubtedly going to be controversial, and it will inevitably raise questions about whether taxpayers in general, rather than the poor, should bear the cost of extending coverage.

But I am prepared, for the sake of discussion, to accept the medicaid budget constraint as Oregon sees it, which means that the state will use a fixed pool of money to care for a medicaid population that will be a bit larger than it is now.

How well does Oregon apply the principle that it has embraced? Not too well, I think.

There are two problems. First Oregon proposes to classify all medical care in 709 categories of diagnosis-treatment pairs. This classification should be compared to the more than 10,000 diagnoses in the *Dictionary of Medical Diagnoses*. The treatability of patients in each of those categories—or at least many of them—is not uniform. Each contains patients who have very good prospective medical outcomes and patients who do not have such good prospective medical outcomes. Therefore, if one wants to combine diagnoses with a reasonably sensitive awareness of the variability of potential outcomes, one is not talking about 10,000 categories, but some multiple of 10,000.

The key point, however, is that 709 categories are far too few to distinguish medically heterogenous situations. Inevitably, some people who receive care will stand to benefit less than some who will be denied care. In short, in any ranking system of this kind, a large overlap will occur in the medical prospects of those who are included and of those who are excluded under the Oregon system.

The second problem is that, apart from a few cases such as AIDS, Oregon makes no allowance for the nature of the medical care provided for a diagnostic category. Not only should we be concerned that each of the multiple of 10,000 diagnostic categories contains patients with similar prospects, but we should also understand that prospects of benefit vary with the intensity of services rendered.

To make sense of a rationing scheme that attempts to allocate resources fairly and efficiently, one must consider not the broad, heterogeneous categories but narrow, homogeneous categories, and one cannot ignore variations in medical therapy that affect the payoff from future care. I think that these considerations are very important because it is virtually certain that if the Oregon Plan is adopted, legitimate and carefully researched reports will soon appear on television, in the newspapers, and on radio revealing that patients who stood to benefit greatly were denied care, while others, who benefited slightly, received it. When that happens, the entire system unravels, and the elected officials who embraced the system will be as far from the television cameras as they can possibly be. A plan that in principle embodies the correct approach to allocating a limited quantity of health care resources will be discredited.

Two responses to my comments are readily apparent. The first is: isn't this system, flawed though it may be, better than what we have? The second is: perhaps in quibbling about the details of the plan, I did not focus on the general principles that have indeed been gotten right.

My answer to that response is twofold. As for the first point, when one tries to do something explicitly, namely, rationing, which may have been done implicitly and sloppily—and identifiable people must assume responsibility for the decisions that have been made— one had better do it right. Those people will have to withstand a lot of criticism on an issue as emotional, divisive, and important as allocating medical resources.

The second point concerning the general principles suggests an analogy. If one were purchasing a new aircraft that had never been flown, and the engineers waved off criticisms of design by saying, "Hey, it's got wings and an engine and a fuselage; don't bother me with calculations of drag and stability and performance in bad weather," one would tell the engineers to go back to the drawing board and report again after they had done their homework properly.

It would be wise for elected officials to beware. If they climb aboard the Oregon plane for a test flight, they will probably go down in political flames. If they insist on a test flight on the Oregon plane, I will not gloat when they crash. But I will try to continue the work that they have bravely, if indiscreetly, begun.

The Political Perspective

Why I Support the Oregon Plan

Over the last twenty years, I have served as director of the Oregon Grey Panthers and as a member of the health and aging committees of the U.S. House of Representatives. In these capacities, I have always sought to protect poor people through mandating benefits, locking them in as a matter of law so that the forces of injustice could not take them away. But it is time to revisit some of our old assumptions about ways of protecting the poor. As a result of this rethinking, I strongly support the Oregon Plan with its revolutionary approach to medicaid.

WHAT'S WRONG?

The medicaid program is at best a crazy quilt of protection. In my state the income eligibility level for medicaid is 50 percent of the federal poverty level. An unmarried mother with two kids and an income of over $5,600 a year is considered too rich for medicaid. A single person or a childless couple in Oregon is out of luck no matter how poor they are. Under today's medicaid program, a poor eight-year-old is ineligible, although a six-year-old sibling would be eligible. In my view, this is irrational and indefensible. We have explicit discriminatory rationing under the medicaid program.

There is also an essential contradiction in our current health care financing and delivery system. On the one hand, some people have no health care coverage at all. These people could not be any worse off under any potential rationing plan than they are now. On the other hand, for people with health insurance, the care possibilities are almost limitless. If you are so inclined, you can be virtually rebuilt physically. You are almost in a position to become technologically immortal.

THE OREGON PLAN

The Oregon Plan seeks to change all this. There are three bills in the Oregon package. One of them, which has received all the coverage, is the part that involves setting priorities. The second part involves establishing a risk pool to cover the uninsurable, an approach often tried in other states.

The third part proposes that, by 1995, all private businesses will have to provide the core package of health benefits for the medicaid population. To their great credit, major business groups in Oregon support applying the standard medicaid package of benefits as a minimum requirement for all businesses in the state of Oregon. At a time when many business groups in this country are "heading for the hills" on the question of mandated benefits because such a program will be too costly, Oregon businesses are saying that they are willing to hitch their health care caboose to the well-being of the poor. That is a very positive development.

Advantages of the Plan

I believe the Oregon Plan is a good idea because I have come to the conclusion that no matter where we are headed in health care—whether toward national health insurance or another solution—we will have to set priorities. We must, as citizens, come together and make some judgments about our preferences.

As a result of an aging population and a technological explosion, we have two inexorable forces at work in health care that will cause expenditures to skyrocket. No matter what approach we use, we will have to make some tough choices. That is why the Oregon exercise of bringing citizens together at more than fifty public hearings across the state and forcing the debate about priorities is so important. Oregon has tackled the difficult task of setting priorities in a sensitive way for over seven hundred conditions and treatments on the ranking list. We have come together, and we have made some choices.

I also think this proposal will be good for poor people. It is currently too easy for politicians to vote against the low-income population. To be sure, we have Representative Henry Waxman and various other members of Congress who have committed themselves to the needs of the poor. Bernie Sanders is also similarly committed. But when most members of Congress vote on health care, they vote on amorphous budgets. They do not vote on real people or on recognizable health services and supplies. They vote to spend $70 billion, $60 billion, $30 billion, whatever the sum is, but it is an abstract sum.

In the state of Oregon that is going to change. We have, in effect, prioritized 709 procedures. Our Health Services Commission has said that more than 600 of them should be funded. The legislature is now going to determine what kind of resources they have for that exercise.*

The point is that when the Oregon legislature votes on that particular measure, it must face real people because everyone under 100 percent of the federal poverty line will know whether the Oregon legislature is voting to grant or deny him or her a basic package of benefits. It will personalize the health care debate and, particularly, the rights of the poor, unlike anything we have ever done in this country. Poor people can say to people in politics, "You voted no on the Oregon medicaid funding program. And, under that Oregon medicaid funding program, I would have received this core package of benefits." It is very exciting to see how the Oregon Plan empowers poor people and gives them additional influence in the political process.

Consumer Protection

Because of the controversy over health care rationing, there must be four consumer protections for this proposal to have a good chance of being approved in Washington.

Initially, there must be a significant amount of additional state revenue for this proposal. We cannot include a large number of additional eligibles—in our state it may be approximately 100,000—and make this budget neutral. The state must find a large amount of additional revenue to help the poor. The sums that are being discussed are between $30 million and $40 million a year.† As many of you know, the federal medicaid program matches those funds on almost a two-to-one basis. Therefore, it is essential that the state bring additional money to the table. Then, for any mandated benefit that is waived, there must be a public hearing so that there is specific oppor-

*The legislature voted to cover services to number 587 [eds.].
†The legislature ultimately approved $33 million in new state funding [eds.].

tunity for discussion. In addition, the secretary of the Department of Health and Human Services would have the right to revoke the waiver at any time that he considered the core package of benefits inadequate for the needs of the poor. Finally, this would be an Oregon-only experiment. Oregon has initiated a program that it ought to be allowed to try. Oregonians are not so naive as to think that this does not have national implications, but Oregon should have an opportunity to attempt this as a five-year demonstration project.

CONCLUSION

There has been a great deal of mythology about what the Oregon Plan seeks to do. The Oregon Plan means different things to different people. If a person is on the classic conservative side of the political spectrum, rationing might be appealing in that dollars taken from skyrocketing health care expenditures will save government money on the poor. If a person is on the other side of the political spectrum, he or she might also believe this is a way to expand access to health care, to cover more poor people, to get additional resources into the system, and, perhaps, most attractively, to ensure that everyone in this country receives the same basic health care plan. This is exactly what the Oregon Plan does. And that is why, with the consumer protections I have outlined, the Oregon proposal has been endorsed by a statewide coalition of approximately ninety labor, consumer, senior, and health groups. I enthusiastically support the Oregon Plan.

BERNARD SANDERS

A National Health Care Alternative to the Oregon Plan

Because the issue of a national health care plan has been of great concern to me as a representative of the state of Vermont, I am delighted to have an opportunity to address this problem. National health care legislation is under consideration that would grant every person in our country all the health care he or she needs without costing more than the $740 billion that is currently being spent.

It is important to place into context the increasing discussion about rationing health care. It must be considered within the framework of what is happening in this country today, as well as during the last ten or fifteen years. The overall economic reality of the country cannot be dismissed when attention turns to health care.

What is happening in this country when we say that if you are rich, you get the best health care in the world; if you are middle class, the level of care is fairly good—but it may not be possible to go to the doctor or hospital all the time; and if you are poor, you might die because society has decided that this treatment is unavailable to you, although it is available for the rich? To a great extent, this reflects the current situation.

During the last ten or fifteen years, a widening gap has been developing between the rich and the poor. One percent of the U.S. population owns one-third of the wealth. We have seen increasing numbers of millionaires and billionaires and the collapse of the middle class, whose workers today make significantly less than they did twenty years ago, in terms of real dollars. That is what is going on.

Therefore, we cannot examine only health care in this discussion. The same thing is happening in education. Millions of working-class students cannot afford to go to college. It is happening in housing, with two million people sleeping on the street. That is the context in which we begin to explain, quite openly, "If you are rich you get one type of care, and if you are middle class, you get another type of care."

I disagree with the Oregon Plan, and I think the plan that we will be developing in Vermont will be a far saner and more humane plan—in fact, a far more efficient plan. But it should be said in support of our friends in Oregon, which has a long tradition of being a progressive state, that what they have done took courage because we must dismiss this notion that there is no rationing in America. Oregon should be commended for at least having the gumption to declare that in all fifty states of the union, including Oregon and Vermont, there is rationing. The current rationing, however, is not done openly. It is not done in serious debate. It is done according to what a person is able to afford. If you have the money, there is no problem. If you do not have the money and are among the 37 million Americans without health insurance, there is rationing. If you are among the 60 million with only partial insurance, there is rationing. Therefore, Oregon must be applauded for at least initiating this discussion.

Vermonters intend to do it differently. There are several reasons that I oppose the Oregon Plan and think the plan I will be proposing, which many Vermonters approve, makes much more sense.

It seems to me that before we talk about rationing, we have to realize that there are only two nations in the entire industrialized world without some kind of national health care system—the United States and South Africa. We must realize that, whereas our system exists in a state of collapse, with large numbers of people lacking any insurance and very high rates of infant mortality and low-weight babies, many countries have a greater longevity and better infant health rates.

Within this context, what can we make of the idea that we are not spending enough money? Is the problem that we are really just too cheap? Are the Canadians, the English, the Swedes, the Europeans, the Japanese, and the Australians just spending a lot more per capita?

Before there is any more insane talk about rationing, we must first understand that the United States spends far more per capita than any other nation on earth. The Canadians are capable of providing basic health care to all of their people, while spending 30 percent less per capita on health care than we do.

So, before we debate whether we give a low-income child a kidney transplant, as opposed to putting money into prenatal care for low-income women, we must ask ourselves the reason that we continue to support a chaotic health care system that allows for 1,500 separate, private insurance providers that, according to a recent study, manage to waste more than $100 billion in billing practices, in bureaucracy, in marketing expenses, and in profit-taking.

My belief is that before we set the poor against the middle class, we must have the political courage to begin to acknowledge that when millions of our people have no health insurance and when we talk about rationing, we have to move toward a single-payer system, eliminate the billing, the profits, and the bureaucracy, and save $100 billion. According to that recent study, the estimate is that such a move could save $1.2 billion in Oregon. Take the money from paper pushing, billing, and profits, and direct it toward health care. Then, we could insure every one of the uninsured people and provide quality health care for all. In my state of Vermont, the numbers are smaller. It is an estimated $200 million. Therefore, before we talk about rationing, we should talk about taking on the drug companies, the insurance companies, the medical equipment suppliers, and the American Medical Association—all of whom are today making billions of dollars from a chaotic system that is disintegrating.

In my view, we do not really have a health care crisis. What we have is a political crisis. We have, increasingly, as many of you know, a one-party system in which the differences between the two major parties are becoming negligible. Throughout the world—in Canada twenty years ago—people had the courage to stand up to the medical-industrial complex. It does not seem that in our country, given the present political leadership, there is the will to do that. So, let me simply say that I do not support, nor will be part of, resuscitating the present system.

Eventually, this issue will lead to more than the debate on kidney transplants. It will go deeper than that unless we are able to develop a national health care system. The present system means walking into a hospital and seeing the rich, who will receive the best care in the world, the middle class, who might receive some care, and triage for the poor, who will die while the rich will live. That is not the system that I will support.

If we have the political will—and, on this issue, the people of this country seem to be far ahead of Congress or the White House; I know the people of my state are—we can stand up to the private insurance companies, the AMA, and the drug companies. The people are prepared to ask why prescription drugs, manufactured in the United

States, are sold at a far higher price here than in Europe or in Canada. They are prepared to ask why certain physicians can make millions of dollars a year in income. Our people are prepared to ask those questions before we live with the status quo and then say, "Gee, there just isn't enough money available. Some will have to die, while others live."

The bottom line is that if we move toward a national health care system, we can save more than $100 billion a year. We can have quality health care for all our people by removing much of the waste that the present system now encourages.

That is the type of proposal that I will present to Congress. It is the type of proposal that I hope the state of Vermont will adopt.

Physician Perspectives

JOHN LA PUMA

Quality-Adjusted Life-Years: Why Physicians Should Reject Oregon's Plan

Robert Kaplan and Michael Garland have explained the primary methodology used to rank services in Oregon. They have touched on some of the technical and philosophical limitations of the methodology. As a practicing internist and clinical ethicist, I would simply like to add some practical, medical limitations of the Oregon Plan's methodology.

It is important to say that the methodology is the heart of the work. Serious clinical ethical questions have been raised about the Oregon methodology, which uses a ranking scheme called a quality-of-well-being scale that is similar to quality-adjusted life-years (QALYs).[1] Rationing health care with QALYs now seems reasonable to many thoughtful people, but it actually will serve to deny medically necessary services to those who are most vulnerable—the medically indigent, especially women and children.

QALYs have several clear benefits. QALYs attempt to clarify judgments about quality of life. As a cost-utility analysis, QALYs may be helpful to policymakers. QALYs may improve the efficiency and objectivity of medical decisionmaking, which would reduce the subjectivity of judgments about quality of life.[2] Finally, QALYs are a potential result of community medical ethics—the public identification,

This paper has been adapted from John La Puma and Edward Lawlor, "Quality Adjusted Life-Years: Ethical Implications for Clinicians and Policymakers," *Journal of the American Medical Association*, vol. 263 (June 6, 1990), pp. 2917–21 (copyright 1990, American Medical Association); and from John La Puma, "Quality Adjusted Life-Years: Ethical Implications and the Oregon Plan," *Issues in Law and Medicine* (forthcoming). The work was supported in part by the American College of Physicians, Lutheran General Hospital, and the Lutheran General Medical Group.

prioritization, and implementation of an equitable, virtuous distribution of health care resources.

Unfortunately, the reintroduction of the Oregon ranking of 709 services ratifies a new financial ethos in medical care. The actuarial study shows that going down just to number 587 on the list would cost an extra $30 million in state spending. This will cover most of what Oregon calls "essential services," and "very important" services, and virtually no "services valuable to certain individuals." Indigent patients will not receive medicine for cerebral hemorrhage in newborns (687 of 709), for gallstones (681 of 709), or for Lou Gehrig's disease (609 of 709). Currently, using QALYs for health policy decisions is problematic and, indeed, unsafe.

QALYS AND MEDICAL ETHICS

The debate about Oregon's use of QALYs occurs on four levels. First, the ranking and funding of health care services balances costs and benefits of the service for the state—not for the patient, or for his or her individual circumstances. Second, doctors will be asked to practice two-tier medicine explicitly. Patients with resources will receive some beneficial treatments, and medicaid patients will receive fewer beneficial treatments. Third, managed-care plans that will provide services to patients may actually profit by manipulating payments, by misusing quality and utilization management, and by rationing services themselves through inconvenience for patients.[3] Fourth, it is assumed that rationing will save money, although the costs of *not* providing care will not be assessed. These costs include intangibles (such as the bad press engendered by seven-year-old Coby Howard's untreated leukemia) and tangibles (Coby's lost lifetime of wages).[4] If the Oregon Plan is fully funded, an additional $40 million in state funding will be needed.[5]

QALYs' Ethical Assumptions

The formal use of QALYs makes six ethical assumptions. First, quality of life can be accurately measured and should have "standing" in determining resource allocation. Second, utilitarianism ("the greatest good for the greatest number") is the appropriate ethical theory for resolving resource allocation dilemmas. Third, equity and efficiency are compatible and should be balanced in QALY construction. Fourth, projections of community preferences for interventions can ethically substitute for the preferences of individual patients when rationing resources. Fifth, older and sicker patients have less "capacity to benefit" from interventions than patients who are younger and healthier. Sixth, doctors will be able to differentiate between a patient's medical need and a resource's availability; will differentiate between being a patient advocate and a public resource agent; will favor the measurable outcome of clinical decisionmaking more than the less measurable process of decisionmaking; and will not use QALYs to make direct clinical decisions. Several of these assumptions are reviewed in more detail here.

Quality of Life

QALYs assume that quality of life can be measured well enough to make policy judgments about it. Some patients with "poor quality of life," however, are unable to make health care decisions and have no one to speak reliably for them; other patients would rather live, regardless of what others think.

One patient at Lutheran General Hospital, Mrs. G., a sixty-nine-year-old woman with severe liver failure, had begun to throw up blood once every three to six weeks and would then lapse into a coma from hepatic encephalopathy. She was on medicaid, lived in a nursing home, was widowed, and had two children with whom she was in regular contact but who lived in another state. She was so sick that whenever she threw up blood it seemed as though she would die, and she was always taken directly to the hospital. The second time this happened, a physician-in-training asked, "Should we continue to treat her?" After she received fluids, medication, and transfusions, she told us on the third hospital day, "It's like a dream when I pass out. I wake up in the hospital, and I feel better. I don't even remember throwing up, and then you treat me, and I go back home." She lived eight more months in this cycle, to her own satisfaction. The lives of patients like Mrs. G.—the indigent, the critically ill, and the elderly— QALYs judge to be of inadequate worth; for groups of patients similar to her, who are *not* asked about their quality of life, quality-of-life assessments cannot be accurately assessed.

The Greatest Good for the Greatest Number, According to the Fewest

Oregon has made an attempt to assess community preferences by holding town meetings before drafting its legislation, but it is well documented that the poor, the elderly, and children generally did not participate in these meetings.[6] It is precisely these groups, however, that will be most affected by the Oregon Plan.

QALYs and the Oregon Plan are controversial not only for what they are but also for the new financial ethos they represent: both are symbolic of a public policy movement to make the delivery of health care a commodity, and to create a businessperson-customer relationship from the doctor-patient relationship. In the current era of cost containment, the physician should not be placed in the position of defending a public policy that is more interested in saving money than in providing medically necessary services. Choosing between being a public agent or a patient advocate is an increasingly clear, yet untenable, choice for physicians.[7]

Whose Autonomy? Whose Justice?

QALYs would project community preferences based on hypothetical medical situations over the preferences of individual patients. An assessment of preferences for an individual medicaid patient in Oregon comes from the preferences of a selected average member of the public—not from the average patient, or from the patient himself or herself. Neither good patient care nor good public health supports this generalization. Rationing in Oregon will not be individualized for individual patients but will be based on a selected sample of the population, despite individual patient circumstances.

Clinical Decisionmaking

Unfortunately, doctors and hospitals may use QALYs as they have used diagnosis-related groups—as direct, clinical decisionmaking tools. Combining equations of efficiency with the need to contain health care costs, however, yields a blunt, economically driven tool. Whether QALYs will be used as clinical maxims, and will therefore override physicians' moral obligations to appeal economic constraints and to provide services that are not reimbursed but are medically necessary, remains to be seen.

The process of clinical decisionmaking is also not taken into account by QALYs. The significance of this criticism is undervalued. Many interactions between doctor and patient do not result in a tangible intervention or in easily measurable data. Patients often seek medical attention for information, reassurance, encouragement, and permission, not only for prescriptions and procedures. Valid, reliable assessments of clinical processes should be undertaken, and they should be as carefully considered as the assessment of outcome. In QALY calculation, there is no attempt to integrate the therapeutic process and outcome of talking with patients or their families.[8]

Finally, can doctors and hospitals differentiate between what is medically needed and what is medically available? Whether the physician's role must be redefined to include "negotiator" and "advocate" at the policy level is the real question. Conserving society's resources has been secondary or tertiary; if such conservation is brought about by considering some patients expendable, especially medically indigent patients, or by serving opposing masters of patient and payer, the seemingly imminent role of public resource agent must be acknowledged, appealed, and refuted.[9]

CONCLUSION

For the Oregon Plan, significant ethical dilemmas of equity, justice, autonomy, beneficence, and discrimination make QALY use unsafe and unwise.

Alternatives to rationing and the use of QALYs exist. They include an emphasis on disease prevention and health promotion, the use of financial disincentives for medical entrepreneurs, a role for primary care physicians in deciding specialist referrals, a willingness to evaluate critically the process and outcome of what we do every day, and a concern for teaching the practice of medical ethics.[10]

If physicians use QALYs to determine which of their patients will receive treatment, full disclosure will not help.[11] Physicians may say to their patients that Oregon does not pay for a needed treatment, but because this information may be insufficient or poorly understood, patients will need independent advice and advocacy. Otherwise, patients' preferences and needs for health care will be replaced by an economic analysis that relies on selected community opinions. Financial criteria should not decide which one of two patients to treat when medical resources exist to treat both patients.[12] Physicians' social responsibility to use resources carefully may supplant their professional responsibility to care for their patients medically.

Available resources should not be used for researching or deploying QALYs, but for different, more fundamental changes in the health care system. Patients go to doctors for help; doctors should not be compelled to refuse medically necessary, appropriate services to patients who would have received their help before Oregon's rationing and who need help now.

NOTES

1. Paul Menzel, *Medical Costs, Moral Choices* (Yale University Press, 1983), pp. 185–95; Alan Maynard and J. B. Devlin, "Economists v. Clinicians: The Crucial Debate," *Health and Social Service Journal*, July 18, 1985, pp. 7–8; R. J. Jarret, "Economics of Coronary Artery Bypass Grafting," *British Medical Journal*, vol. 291 (August 31, 1985), p. 600; Alwyn Smith, "Qualms about Qalys," *Lancet*, vol. 8542 (May 16, 1987), pp. 1134–36; John Harris, "QALYfying the Value of Life," *Journal of Medical Ethics*, vol. 13 (September 1987), pp. 117–23; *The Ian Ramsey Centre Working Party Report on Decision-Making and Quality of Life* (Oxford University, St. Cross College, 1989); and John Rawles, "Castigating QALYs," *Journal of Medical Ethics*, vol. 15 (September 1989), pp. 143–47.

2. James A. Kruse, Mary C. Thill-Baharozian, and Richard W. Carlson, "Comparison of Clinical Assessment with APACHE II for Predicting Mortality Risk in Patients Admitted to a Medical Intensive Care Unit," *Journal of the American Medical Association*, vol. 260 (September 23–30, 1988), pp. 1739–42.

3. Gerald W. Grumet, "Health Care Rationing through Inconvenience: The Third Party's Secret Weapon," *New England Journal of Medicine*, vol. 321 (August 31, 1989), pp. 607–11.

4. David M. Eddy, "What's Going on in Oregon?" *Journal of the American Medical Association*, vol. 266 (July 17, 1991), pp. 417–21.

5. Timothy Egan, "Oregon Shakes Up Pioneering Health Plan for the Poor," *New York Times*, February 22, 1991.

6. Susan Adelman, "How to Approach the Issue of Rationing Care," *American Medical News*, January 21, 1991, p. 23.

7. Frederick Abrams, "Patient Advocate or Secret Agent," *Journal of the American Medical Association*, vol. 256 (October 3, 1986), pp. 1784–85.

8. Eric Cassell, *Talking with Patients*, vol. 2: *Clinical Technique* (MIT Press, 1985).

9. Douglas F. Levinson, "Toward Full Disclosure of Referral Restrictions and Financial Incentives by Prepaid Health Plans," *New England Journal of Medicine*, vol. 317 (December 31, 1987), pp. 1729–31; Michael Reagan, "Physicians as Gatekeepers: A Complex Challenge," ibid., pp. 1731–34; Alan Hillman, "Financial Incentives for Physicians in HMOs: Is There a Conflict of Interest?" ibid., pp. 1743–48; and John La Puma, Christine Cassel, and Holly Humphrey, "Ethics, Economics, and Endocarditis: The Physician's Role in Resource Allocation," *Archives of Internal Medicine*, vol. 148 (August 1988), pp. 1809–11.

10. Arnold Relman, "The Trouble with Rationing," *New England Journal of Medicine*, vol. 323 (September 27, 1990), pp. 911–13; and Norman Levinsky, "Age as a Criterion for Rationing Health Care," *New England Journal of Medicine*, vol. 322 (June 21, 1990), pp. 1813–16.

11. Marc A. Rodwin, "Physicians' Conflicts of Interest—The Limitations of Disclosure," *New England Journal of Medicine*, vol. 321 (November 16, 1989), pp. 1405–08.

12. Robert Steinbrook and Bernard Lo, "The Oregon Medicaid Project—Will It Provide Adequate Care?" *New England Journal of Medicine*, vol. 326 (January 30, 1992), pp. 340–44.

STEPHEN M. AYRES

Rationality, Not Rationing, in Health Care

The inquiry into whether to ration health care to poor people in American society must first begin with an assessment of health care at the end of the twentieth century and the reason it is in such scarce supply that it must be rationed. It is difficult to conceive of a shortage of health care resources when our newspapers and television screens are full of glittering reports about the latest miracle drug, and every hospital, large or small, is promoted as a major medical center. Health care itself is not in short supply, but the money to pay for it is.

The promise of health care has been fulfilled in large measure, and the results are truly amazing. Today, 71 percent of Americans can expect to live to the age of seventy; only 32 percent could reach that age in 1900.[1] Much of this improvement in health status can be attributed to the almost exponential growth of scientific knowledge and the ability to apply that knowledge to the maintenance of health and the treatment of disease. This increase in survivorship has been almost linear and was achieved for much of the century without much increase in cost. The acceleration of health costs began in the late 1960s as per capita total health expenditures (real dollars) in the United States rose from $346 per American in 1970 to $2,124 in 1988 and to more than $3,000 in 1991.[2] It is projected to rise to more than $5,000 by the year 2000.

The problem is not the availability of financial resources for the purchase of health care but the distribution of those resources. Although the fruits of biomedical science have led to improved life expectancy for many, the benefits of medicine have not been universally experienced. Seventy-eight percent of white women will live at least to seventy, but only 47 percent of black men will reach that age. Eight percent of white male deaths and 12 percent of black male deaths result from accidental or intentional violence; the remaining deaths among both whites and blacks result primarily from heart disease, cancer, and stroke. Access to those resources that permit living to at least the biblical three score and ten has been denied to one group of individuals, which demonstrates the consequences of rationing health care for those with the poorest health status and the least ability to pay. Can anyone believe that this sort of rationing is consistent with the foundations of American democracy?

Health care has always been an important public policy issue in this country, but the nature of the dialogue has shifted from that of the 1960s, when the main concern was access. The problems of access became so devastating that the discussion rapidly moved from the level of polite conversation to the burning of cities. Newark exploded when the New Jersey College of Medicine moved from Jersey City into the heart of the Newark ghetto. The "taking of 150 acres therefore meant something to different people—a necessity to some, a threat to others. So the medical school—to a degree unwittingly and innocently and to a degree wittingly and, I think, not so innocently—became the lightning rod of discontent and one of the declared causes of the revolution in Newark."[3] In the wake of riots, which developed largely over the issue of access to health care, the National Advisory Committee on Civil Disorders (the Kerner Commission) concluded that the main cause of the riots was pervasive racism and segregation, which results in "the continuing exclusion of great numbers of Negroes from the benefits of economic progress through discrimination in employment and education, and their enforced confinement in segregated housing and schools. The corrosive and degrading effects of this condition and the attitudes that underlie it are the source of the deepest bitterness and at the center of the problem of racial disorder."[4] The report noted that "poverty means deficient diets, lack of medical care, inadequate shelter and clothing, and often lack of awareness of potential health needs. As a result, about 30 percent of all persons with family incomes less than $2,000 per year suffer from chronic health problems which adversely affect their employment." Today, the health status in the ghetto is worse, not better, but the discussion is about rationing rather than access and quality care.

Unlike health costs in most developed countries in the world, health costs in the United States are met by different government and private sources. Private sources provided $351 billion in 1989; taxes to state and federal governments provided $253 billion. Medicare costs were $102 billion, and medicaid costs paid by both state and federal governments totaled $64 billion.[5] Because health premiums paid by employers are fully deductible from federal taxes, the more than $50–$60 billion currently lost by the federal government represents a large subsidy to many of the employed population.[6] Thus, federal support of health care costs goes to the elderly and the employed, while the unemployed and underemployed receive less than 20 percent of the total federal subsidy. Despite the generally acknowledged evidence that poor people are sicker than the more affluent (the socioeconomic gradient), the proportion of poor Americans enrolled in medicaid fell from 63 to 46 percent between 1975 and 1983.[7] Most discussions of rationing today have dealt with the control of these medicaid costs. They have, however, generally exempted consideration of the other much larger costs. This marked unevenness in the distribution of medical resources creates what Morreim has called "a stratified scarcity."[8]

The improvement in health status revealed in survival statistics is the result of advances in the physical, chemical, biomedical, and social sciences. But the mathematically exponential growth in health care costs leads to the important question whether life to the longest possible age is one of the "inalienable rights of life, liberty, and the pursuit of happiness" specified in the Declaration of Independence. Much of the increase in life expectancy is due to the general availability of effective, but expensive, medical technology. The cost of modern care, however, may well be greater than necessary, and probably many of the methods used to save lives may not necessarily ensure that survivors have a reasonable quality of life. The biomedical sciences have achieved a level of success that has challenged the social and political sciences. American thought must now turn to an examination of the level of health status necessary for happiness and the obvious discussion of the importance of health status in the group of weighted trade-offs (housing, food, transportation, education, employment, a healthful environment, national security) that create what is called happiness. The discussion must also include a candid acknowledgement that the United States is the only country in the developed world that does not provide health care for all its citizens.[9] The absence of such universal coverage is even more shocking when one realizes that most of the developing countries, poor as they are, still manage to provide health care for all.

SHOULD HEALTH CARE BE RATIONED
FOR SOME AMERICANS?

Many Americans remember food rationing during World War II as a sacrifice made willingly by the entire population. The suggestion has now been made that health care be rationed for some Americans. The consideration of rationing health care to those unable to pay for it seems evidence of a health care system totally beyond control. The inability to develop a coherent American health policy is a result primarily of an ingrained national mistrust of rational thinking; it is part of the larger failure to cope with the human management of science and technology. These two separate cultures—science and nonscience—move forward in strikingly different ways. The acquisition of new scientific information advances dramatically in what must be considered an exponential manner. The societal response to news about human evolution, environmental contamination, or the appearance and spread of the human immunodeficiency virus is reserved, suspicious, and even hostile. In consequence, after periods of little change, cyclical sea-shifts in culture appear as scientific theory is attacked by one group and defended by another. The American Right at this moment attacks persons who become infected with HIV; the American Left sees conspiracy in environmental and occupational spoliation. Each interprets science in terms of its own bias.

The national debate over the cost of health care and the nearly universal perception that a cohesive national health policy must be formulated are evidence of the discontinuity between science and human affairs. Although medical science has advanced exponentially, the ability to cope with its success has varied widely and cyclically. Retirement pensions under a social security plan were approved in 1935, and parallel recommendations for health insurance were also made. There was considerable optimism for passage; Arthur Schlesinger quotes Harry Hopkins as saying that "with one bold stroke we could carry the American people with us, not only for unemployment insurance but for sickness and health insurance." Vigorous pressure from the American Medical Association, however, defeated the bill.[10] In his memoirs President Harry Truman described his attempt to introduce legislation for National Health Insurance in 1949, but, he said, it was opposed by "reactionaries and leaders of 'organized medicine.' The same false charge of 'socialized medicine' was used to discredit the program and to confuse and mislead the people."[11] A health insurance program for the elderly (medicare) was given the highest priority among President Lyndon Johnson's Great Society programs and was voted into law in 1964. Although it was approved at the same time, medicaid was considered a public assistance bill; therefore, it never received the popular support afforded medicare. Whereas national standards were required for medicare, medicaid standards and funding levels were left to the states. Support for medicaid has gradually collapsed. Most recently, John Kitzhaber, president of the Oregon State Senate and an emergency medicine physician, proposed a unique and radical method for containing a small portion of expenditures for health—the medicaid program.[12]

DISTRIBUTE HEALTH RESOURCES ON THE BASIS OF BENEFIT

What are the implications of what Oregon has considered to be a "Healthier Approach to Health Care"[13] and others have thought to be "Oregon's Bold Mistake"?[14] Although the words *ration* and *rational* are both derived from the same Latin stem meaning *to reason*, they have acquired far different meanings in current American parlance. Rationing suggests the limitation of some substance or service, while rational means an intelligent way of approaching a specific problem. There certainly is no shortage of health care resources in the United States, and the country's position as the number-one health care spender in the world suggests there are sufficient financial resources. Because these financial and health care resources appear to be inappropriately distributed, common sense would suggest that a rational approach to the development of health care policy would make rationing unnecessary. A rational approach might suggest that a specific health intervention is useful or effective if it produces an obvious benefit. The effectiveness of an intervention is not absolute, however, but is relative to the specific clinical situation in which it is used. Thus, some people could clearly benefit from a given course of action, while others could not. A rational health policy would not limit a given intervention to special groups such as the wealthy; it would limit its use to those who could benefit from it. The emphasis would be on making it available to those who needed it, not on arbitrarily limiting its use.

The good physician has always prescribed diagnostic and therapeutic interventions on the basis of usefulness, probably unaware that Jeremy Bentham defined utility as "that property in any object, whereby it tends to produce benefit, advantage, pleasure, good or happiness" at a time when medicine was still in the dark ages.[15] Paul Ellwood introduced the idea of benefit or utility to the health policy field as "outcomes management."[16] William Roper and others collapsed the qualities of medical effectiveness and medical appropriateness into the term "effectiveness."[17]

The weakness of any system that attempts to limit the availability of medical interventions on the basis of age, race, financial status, or effectiveness is that guidelines or "parameters" can only define usefulness in an abstract sense—not prescribe whether a given intervention might be useful for a specific patient. The patient himself is a poor purchaser of health services; even the most knowledgeable of them all—the sick physician—is reputed to be the most difficult of patients. Choosing an effective intervention for the appropriate patient is complicated by the incredibly perverse economic incentives contained in the health insurance system. Health insurance began as a hospital insurance program, and physicians and their patients quickly discovered that an uncovered diagnostic procedure such as a gastrointestinal X ray could be covered if the physician recommended hospital admission and the patient agreed that he had enough abdominal discomfort to justify such a course of action.

THE PERSONAL PHYSICIAN AS PATIENT ADVOCATE AND GATEKEEPER

Caveat emptor is an almost empty phrase in a medical marketplace that is filled with glittering statements of perfection, which suggest that every hospital able to create a commercial message is a modern temple of healing! Who can lead either the healthy or the ill through the confusing web of those who would profit from their ignorance? The obvious answer, known from the dim past well before the time of Hippocrates, is the personal physician.

Any health care system must begin with the primary care physician and a group of individuals—the well, the ill, and the worried well. The personal physician is presumably one who has little financial incentive for selecting an inappropriate intervention; he is therefore probably best suited to the role of gatekeeper. Representatives from insurance companies are employed to restrain health costs; specialist physicians are justifiably enthusiastic about their own areas of expertise and view potential patients as important opportunities to exercise their skills. The primary care physician may sometimes select a specialist to perform certain tasks that would add to the length of the poorly reimbursed primary care visit, but he or she is usually protected from direct financial temptations by the prohibition of fee splitting. Hospital-provided offices at low rent and in close proximity to specialists could encourage inappropriate referral to specialists, but there is little direct information about whether such inappropriate behavior actually occurs. In contrast, regular visits for health assessment at reasonable intervals, an understanding of a person's health status and social environment, and the ability to consult with reliable specialty consultants allow the personal physician to provide appropriate care for what is aptly called "the whole person." The physician presumably understands the value systems held by the patient and his family; he is therefore in the best position to develop a diagnostic and therapeutic approach that balances benefit, risk, burden, and cost.

Half of the physicians in England, for example, are primary care physicians. They account for more than 80 percent of health visits but only 20 percent of health costs.[18] Their continuing relationship with their patients leads to decreased hospitalization and use of specialty care. Such continuity of care is particularly important for impoverished groups, and there is reliable evidence that regular association with a primary care physician can improve health status among those groups of people.

The personal physician is at the vortex of conflicts over the costs of health care; these conflicts are particularly burdensome if the physician practices in either rural or inner-city locations. Centuries of medical practice rooted in the ethics of the Judeo-Christian tradition have emphasized the exemplar role of the Good Samaritan embodied in the family physician. Legal precedents, which support this charitable function, suggest that a physician must deliver the same standard of care to all patients, regardless of their ability to pay. If physicians do not use state-of-the-art diagnostic and therapeutic modalities in the care of their patients, and if they abandon them because the patients have no more money, they may be guilty of negligence.

BEYOND THE OREGON APPROACH

The Oregon initiative demonstrates the importance of state leadership and is consistent with Rashi Fein's statement that "we cannot solve either the access or the cost problem by itself. The enactment of legislation to attain one goal (but not both) would prove to be an unstable 'solution.' "[19] Oregon chose to increase the number of medicaid beneficiaries and to control cost by managing and limiting the services available to the expanded medicaid group. States have the authority to regulate health insurers and some—New York and Massachusetts, for example—have used this power to develop proposed health care systems that would offer universal access to all the state's citizens. Medicaid recipients in thirty-three states are enrolled in managed-care programs designed to control costs. The American Medical Association has agreed that "it is no longer acceptable morally, ethically, or economically for so many of our people to be medically uninsured or seriously underinsured" and has devoted an entire issue of its journal to a discussion of thirteen separate proposals for health care reform.[20] Such vigorous activity by national policymakers gains added impetus from the realization that many newer scientific contributions may not be as inflationary as present-day technology and may actually decrease health care costs. Prevention of AIDS, coronary artery disease, and high blood pressure by new pharmacologic techniques, for example, could substantially reduce dependence on long hospitalizations and expensive surgical procedures.

Development of a basic benefits plan, which includes preventive care and diagnosis and treatment for illness and injury, is a natural evolution of the health policy experiments proposed by Oregon, New York, and Massachusetts. The federal government should require that all Americans have access to the basic benefits plan so that individual insurers can be encouraged to compete in the areas of quality and cost but not on the scope of coverage. The primary care physician, in consultation with specialty physicians where indicated, should be the gatekeeper and should be empowered to use these beneficial diagnostic or therapeutic measures without other forms of authorization. Their actions, however, would be compared with national or state norms during a yearly analysis of activities, which could also include the total health care costs attributable to the patients in their practice.

Much of the present American health care system is funded through tax-exempt premiums that purchase employer-sponsored health benefit packages. Self-employed persons are exempt from only 25 percent of the cost of health care insurance, but all costs for employer-sponsored plans are borne by pretax dollars. Small-business employers are often unable to provide health insurance, and their employees may remain uninsured. Unemployment leads to loss of health benefits, and job mobility is reduced by a job-related system. An important "new" idea is that responsibility for obtaining health care insurance be given to individuals and families rather than to employers, and that tax-credits related to annual income be used for financing such insurance.[21] Only the basic benefits package should be funded by either tax credits or tax exemptions. People seeking expanded health insurance for interventions that are not included in the basic benefits package could obtain coverage, but payment for that coverage would not be exempt from taxation. This reduction in tax-exempt revenues would provide an immediate source of revenue that could be used to make the basic benefits package available to all Americans. Managed or coordinated care would be encouraged by allowing insurers to negotiate with hospitals and physician groups in what Alain Enthoven and Richard Kronick have called "managed competition."[22] Efficiencies in care delivery and charges that are indexed to volume could provide incentives for constraining costs without limiting quality or access.

It may seem predictable for a medical educator to advocate returning the control of health care decisions to the patient and his or her physician, but there really is no other way. Health care by megacorporation, computer, or bureaucrat simply will not work. Young physicians today seem much more socially responsible than some of their predecessors and could be readily educated into the ways of a reformed health care system if they believed in the equity of that system. Indeed, a recent survey of resident physicians demonstrated their general willingness to participate in a government-funded national health insurance program even though they preferred fee-for-service health care.[23] While Americans herald their ingenuity, the time is at hand to admit that the European countries have long outperformed us in health care matters.

More than 2,300 years ago, Plato warned his colleagues about the danger of creating two separate classes of patients and physicians. The Athenian in conversation with a Spartan and a Cretan observes that

> there are two classes of doctors. And did you ever observe that there are two classes of patients in states, slaves and freemen; and the slave doctors run about and cure slaves, or wait for them in their dispensaries—practitioners of this sort never talk to their patients individually, or let them talk about their own individual complaints. The slave-doctor prescribes what mere experience suggests, as if he had exact knowledge; and when he has given his orders, like a tyrant, he rushes off with equal assurance to some other servant who is ill. . . . But the other doctor, who is a freeman, attends and practices upon freemen; and he carries his enquiries far back, and goes into the nature of the disorder; he enters into discourse with the patient and with his friends, and is at once getting information from the sick man, and also instructing him as far as he is able, and he will not prescribe for him until he has first convinced him; at last when he has brought the patient more and more under his persuasive influences and set him on the road to health, he attempts to effect a cure.[24]

There must be a national health care policy, the system must be reformed, patients must receive care that they need and from which they can benefit, and there must be a single level of access and delivery of health care. The more than $700 billion of current health care costs must be reallocated in a rational way without arbitrary rationing. And there must be neither slaves nor slave doctors.

NOTES

1. National Center for Health Statistics, *Vital Statistics of the United States, 1988: Life Tables* (March 1991), p. 12.

2. Katherine Levit and others, "National Health Spending 1989," *Health Affairs*, vol. 10 (Spring 1991), p. 119.

3. Paul Ylvisaker, "What Are the Problems of Health Care Delivery in Newark?" in John Norman, ed., *Medicine in the Ghetto* (Appleton-Century Crofts, 1969), p. 101.

4. *Report of the National Advisory Commission on Civil Disorders* (Bantam Books, 1968), pp. 203, 269.

5. Levit and others, "National Health Spending 1989," p. 123.

6. Mark Pauly and others, "A Plan for 'Responsible National Health Insurance,'" *Health Affairs*, vol. 10 (Spring 1991), pp. 5–25.

7. Robert Blendon and others, "Uncompensated Care by Hospitals or Public Insurance for the Poor: Does It Make a Difference?" *New England Journal of Medicine*, vol. 314 (May 1, 1986), pp. 1160–63.

8. E. Haavi Morreim, "Stratified Scarcity: Redefining the Standard of Care," *Law, Medicine and Health Care*, vol. 17 (Winter 1989), pp. 356–67.

9. Ruth Leger Sivard, *World Military and Social Expenditures, 1989* (Washington: World Priorities, 1989).

10. Arthur M. Schlesinger, Jr., *The Age of Roosevelt*, vol. 2: *The Coming of the New Deal* (Houghton Mifflin, 1959), p. 307.

11. Harry S. Truman, *Years of Trial and Hope, 1946–1952* (Doubleday, 1956), pp. 20–21.

12. John Kitzhaber, "A Healthier Approach to Health Care," *Issues in Science and Technology*, vol. 4 (Winter 1990–91), pp. 59–65.

13. Ibid.

14. Al Gore, Jr., "Oregon's Bold Mistake," *Academic Medicine*, vol. 65 (October 1990), pp. 64–65.

15. Jeremy Bentham, "Introduction to the Principles of Morals and Legislation" (1780), in *Dictionary of the History of Ideas* (Scribner, 1973), vol. 4, p. 450.

16. Paul M. Ellwood, "Shattuck Lecture-Outcome Management: A Technology of Patient Experience," *New England Journal of Medicine*, vol. 318 (June 9, 1988), pp. 1549–56.

17. William L. Roper and others, "Effectiveness in Health Care: An Initiative to Evaluate and Improve Medical Practice," *New England Journal of Medicine*, vol. 319 (November 3, 1988), pp. 1197–1202.

18. Gordon Moore, "Let's Provide Primary Care to All Uninsured Americans—Now!" *Journal of the American Medical Association*, vol. 265 (April 24, 1991), pp. 2108–09.

19. Rashi Fein, "The Health Security Partnership: A Federal State Universal Insurance and Cost-Containment Program," *Journal of the American Medical Association*, vol. 265 (May 15, 1991), pp. 2555–58.

20. George Lundberg, "National Health Care Reform: An Aura of Inevitability Is Upon Us," *Journal of the American Medical Association*, vol. 265 (May 15, 1991), pp. 2565–66.

21. Pauly and others, "Plan for 'Responsible National Health Insurance,'" p. 24.

22. Alain Enthoven and Richard Kronick, "Universal Health Insurance through Incentives Reform," *Journal of the American Medical Association*, vol. 265 (May 15, 1991), pp. 2532–36.

23. Rodney A. Hayward, Richard L. Kravitz, and Martin F. Shapiro, "The U.S. and Canadian Health Care Systems: Views of Resident Physicians," *Annals of Internal Medicine*, vol. 115 (August 15, 1991), pp. 308–14.

24. Plato, "Laws 4," in Benjamin Jowett, tr., *The Dialogues of Plato* (London: Oxford University Press, 1924), ln. 720, p. 103.

ANTHONY P. TARTAGLIA

Is Talk of Rationing Premature?

This paper presents a view from the multitiered perspective of an academic physician, a hematologist, a hospital administrator, a medical college dean, and a member of various regulatory boards in New York State.

Economists, ethicists, and philosophers speak a different language than physicians do. All these groups are going to have to learn to speak the same language. Physicians often get the impression that the ethicists, economists, and philosophers believe they can solve health care problems without physicians. In reality, the latter are essential to whatever solution this country develops for its health care crisis. Everyone, therefore, must be able to communicate effectively.

There are inexorable pressures in this country driving health care costs ever upward. If the health care system is not changed, health care costs can only continue to rise. There are many reasons for this, but an obvious one is the rapidly aging population, which requires more care. In addition, there is an explosion of new technology, which is extremely expensive. New technology probably cannot be suppressed; therefore, there will be increased costs for this technology. Finally, the AIDS epidemic continues unabated and will be an ever-increasing financial drain on our health care system. There are other causes for the pressure forcing up health care costs in the United States, but these three alone would drive health care costs inexorably higher in the years ahead. Therefore, if society determines that there is going to be an upper limit on the amount of money that will be spent for health care, and there are simultaneously irresistible pressures to increase health care costs, then undoubtedly the only solution will be rationing of health care resources.

In this context, it seems worthwhile to examine the Oregon program as an experiment with potentially great implications for this country. The people who contributed to the development of that plan are truly admirable. Indeed, if the U.S. health care system does not change, some form of rationing will be inevitable, but that contingency is extremely troubling. The idea that the health care system will remain the same as it is today should not be true. It ought to be able to change and improve health care delivery before a rationing system becomes necessary.

Traditionally, first-year medical students learn the following approach toward treating a patient. They first ask the patient his or her chief complaint. Then they take a complete history and perform a physical examination. Tests are ordered and a problem list is developed. Based on this problem list, a treatment plan is developed. This is the way physicians traditionally approach their patients; the same approach can be used in analyzing and developing a treatment plan for the health care crisis.

The chief complaint about the health care system is that it costs too much for what it provides. For example, it is often said that the U.S. neonatal mortality rate is much higher than that of other developed nations. Our longevity is no different from that of other industrialized nations. There are 37 million Americans who have either no health care insurance or inadequate health care insurance and, therefore, receive inadequate health care. Yet, health care expenditures were in excess of $700 billion for 1991. I suspect that if we had discovered the Fountain of Youth and everyone could be kept alive and feeling and looking as they did at age twenty, no one would care about the health care costs of this system. This is not the case. As a society, we have decided that the costs of the current system are too great for its value.

Contrary to popular opinion, the U.S. health care system has been examined ad nauseam. Many articles and books have been written about it. Using the chief complaint and the knowledge of the health care system, one does not require genius to develop a problem list and a treatment plan for our health care programs. In fact, it takes so little genius to develop this problem list that I will present one that I have developed myself.

—It is generally agreed that we do not have enough primary care physicians to ensure primary care access for all Americans needing health care. In addition, more and more health care will be provided through managed-care programs and Health Maintenance Organizations (HMOs).

—We must place greater emphasis on preventive care. A phenom-

enal amount of money can be saved in our health care system by disease prevention as opposed to treatment of diseases that have already
developed. All of society must become involved in this preventive
care program. It is not a program that can be effective if it is only
practiced by a few physicians or promulgated by a few organizations.
What kind of preventive care am I talking about? It has been estimated that smoking-related problems cost our health care system
over $65 billion a year. The cessation of smoking would therefore save
enormous sums of money. It has been estimated that a similar amount
of money is spent in our health care system for alcohol-related problems. In addition, billions of dollars are spent each year in caring for
people who have been injured in alcohol-related motor vehicle accidents, and many more billions of dollars are spent caring for people
who have been injured by firearms. If society developed strategies to
control these problems, an enormous amount of money would be
saved.

—Recently published studies by the RAND Corporation noted that
17 percent of all coronary angiography studies were performed inappropriately. Likewise, 17 percent of all upper gastrointestinal endoscopies were also performed for inappropriate reasons. If the category of probably inappropriate is added, then as many as 25 percent
of these procedures were found to be performed for inadequate and
inappropriate reasons. When RAND evaluated carotid endarterec-
tomy, it found that 66 percent of these operations were performed
either for completely inappropriate or probably inappropriate reasons.[1]

In a similar vein, a study done in Massachusetts several years ago
revealed that well over 30 percent of all laboratory testing on patients
in a community hospital was done for inappropriate reasons. Interestingly enough, the authors were able to institute procedures that
effectively eliminated much of the unnecessary testing.[2] If guidelines
were to be developed for the performance of procedures and laboratory tests, a great amount of money would be saved.

—Many things are done in medicine that are believed to be worthwhile and yet have never been tested and proved to be effective. Indeed, many of these procedures and therapies have proved to be ineffective when tested with appropriate research methodologies.
Several examples come to mind. In the 1940s, when an infant was
born with a widened mediastinum, the infant was diagnosed as hav-

ing status thymaticus lympathicus. What a wonderful name. This condition was treated with radiation to the mediastinum. Many years later it was learned that the reason the mediastinum was widened was because the thymus of the infant was enlarged. It was soon learned that radiation was not only not indicated but truly harmful. Indeed, thirty to forty years later, the penalty for this therapy is a higher incidence of carcinoma of the thyroid in the recipients of this radiation treatment.

Years ago, everyone who had more than one sore throat immediately had his tonsils removed. Today, we know that this is not good medicine and try everything possible to prevent tonsillectomies. For a number of years every woman who delivered a child by cesarean section was forevermore committed to having all of her future children by C-section. We now know that this is not necessary and that many women can have subsequent children by the normal vaginal route. Finally, the studies by Dr. Wennberg have demonstrated that there is great diversity in the type of medical care provided for a given medical condition in various areas of the United States.[3] One is now hard pressed to detect any significant difference in outcome despite differences in the medical care provided for many conditions. In summary, a great deal of what we do is done inappropriately and a great deal that we do is ineffective.

—The United States spends a great amount of money on the care of the terminally ill. Our medical intensive care units are filled with people who have irreversible heart and pulmonary disease or irreversible terminal cancer. Yet, these people are subjected to all the technology available in our institutions. The end result of all this therapy is perhaps the prolongation of their lives for several months. We must begin to ask ourselves what value such a limited life has compared with the many years that the person has lived. New societal principles must be developed concerning the care of the terminally ill, the extremely low birth weight neonate, and others. The ethical issues are great, but it is time to look at them honestly and develop new societal mores concerning them.

—A great deal has been said about the Canadian system of health care. It may or may not be the best system around. It is questionable whether it would be appropriate for the United States. The administrative structure of the Canadian health care system, however, is extremely attractive when compared with that of this country. A health care system such as ours that spends twenty-four cents out of every dollar for administration cannot be a good system. In some way, we must develop a more streamlined, cost-effective and cost-efficient administrative system for whatever health care system we develop.

—American medicine is probably the most highly regulated health care system in the world. Indeed, New York State is distinguished by what is probably the most regulated health care system in this country. Behind every regulation there is probably a good intention. When one adds all the regulations together, however, one ends up with a system of micromanagement and strangling regulation that costs a huge amount of money. The regulatory system that has developed in this country should be reviewed and replaced by such other systems as outcome-monitoring quality assurance programs that will both ensure good quality medical care and cost much less.

—Finally, a word about the malpractice system. Our current malpractice system costs more that $9.2 billion a year in premiums for doctors alone.[4] It is unclear what the total cost of the system is in the United States. In addition, it has been demonstrated that there is no significant correlation between those who are injured by malpractice and those who are rewarded by the tort system. A better system of compensation for those persons harmed by negligence must be developed in this country.

This is the problem list that afflicts the health care system. To change this system, a treatment and correction plan must be developed for all elements of the system that need fixing. Frequently, the approach to changes in the health care system has been described as a process of "disjointed incrementalism." We nibble at the periphery of the problem but do not make the fundamental changes required. If we made the changes necessary to correct the problem list that I have described, we would be saving billions upon billions of dollars. Indeed, the savings would probably be so great that there would be no need for rationing at this time.

What is of concern, therefore, is the thought that instead of devoting our collective energies to providing the solutions to the problems that have been outlined, we are merely going to accept the concept that change is impossible and proceed to a rationing program in this country. Formidable forces are very likely arrayed against significant change in our health care system. Among these forces are the doctors themselves, who, despite many problems, continue to do well financially. The lawyers have a vested interest in maintaining our current malpractice system. The insurance companies wish to continue our current system in which there are at least 1,500 different insurance carriers. There is an entire bureaucracy that owes its jobs to our current health care system. So, what can be done? Do we concede as a society that our current health care system cannot change, and because of the inexorable forces leading to escalating costs, do we move toward a rationing system? Or, do we as a society demand that, despite the forces arrayed against change, we unite to develop a cohesive, coherent, and equitable health care policy for our nation? The development of such a comprehensive health care policy requires that all elements of society begin to work collaboratively on the strategies to resolve the problems that plague our current system.

This is the reason I am troubled. My conscience rebels at the thought that we will proceed with an experiment in rationing that will limit some health care to some segments of our society—namely, the poor—while we merrily go on our way unable and unwilling to make the changes in our health care system that would preclude or at least ameliorate the need for rationing.

Therefore, no one should believe that something wonderful in the form of rationing will happen for our people. Instead, we ought to proceed with a new conviction that what is needed at this time is a comprehensive health care policy and strategies to implement it. We should demand that our legislators and elected officials stop playing politics with this issue and unite to develop a comprehensive health care policy. This country is desperately in need of such a policy, and we should demand that one be developed in the very near future.

NOTES

1. Lucian L. Leape and others, "Does Inappropriate Use Explain Small-Area Variations in the Use of Health Care Services?" *Journal of the American Medical Association*, vol. 263 (February 2, 1990), pp. 669–72; and Robert H. Brook and others, "Diagnosis and Treatment of Coronary Disease: Comparison of Doctor's Attitudes in the USA and the UK," *Lancet*, vol. 1 (April 2, 1988), pp. 750–53.

2. Steven L. Gortmaker and others, "A Successful Experiment to Reduce Unnecessary Laboratory Use in a Community Hospital," *Medical Care*, vol. 26 (June 1988), pp. 631–42.

3. John E. Wennberg and others, "Hospital Use and Mortality among Medicare Beneficiaries in Boston and New Haven," *New England Journal of Medicine*, vol. 321 (October 26, 1989), pp. 1168–73; and John E. Wennberg, Jean L. Freeman, and William J. Culp, "Are Hospital Services Rationed in New Haven or Over-Utilized in Boston?" *Lancet*, vol. 1 (May 23, 1987), pp. 1185–89.

4. American Medical Association Board of Trustees, "Report of the Special Task Force on Professional Liability and Insurance and the Advisory Panel on Professional Liability," *Journal of the American Medical Association*, vol. 257 (February 13, 1987), pp. 810–12.

WILLIAM SHOEMAKER, C. BOYD JAMES, ARTHUR W. FLEMING,
EUGENE HARDIN, GARY J. ORDOG, ROSALYN STERLING-SCOTT,
& JONATHAN WASSERBERGER

De Facto Rationing of Emergency Medical Services

The Oregon Plan has provoked debate on whether the United States
should ration health services as a matter of policy and whether it is
fair to single out poor persons to bear the brunt of rationing. To place
this debate in the proper context, the following points should be
made. First, for the poor and the uninsured, there is already a good
deal of health care rationing; moreover, much of that rationing is related to a lack of available resources. Second, the uneven availability
of health insurance coverage has an effect upon hospitals' ability and
willingness to provide care—even to acutely ill patients. Thus, rationing is done partly according to one's ability to pay. Third, many health
care problems are directly embedded in larger social pathologies
(such as drug abuse, gang warfare, and poverty). Therefore, efforts to
solve these health care problems require attacking the broader issues.
To illustrate these points, we consider here the ramifications of rationing in the county hospitals that are primarily responsible for the care
of emergency patients and, in particular, trauma victims.

The impact of rationing on the emergency medical system (EMS)
should be of great interest to society in general. Physical trauma,
which has the most dramatic effect on the EMS, is the leading cause
of death among young people (under forty years of age); affects all
ages, ethnic groups, social strata, and classes; occurs unexpectedly
and, in most instances, when the patient is least prepared financially
and psychologically; is estimated to cost $18 billion annually; and re-
quires an organized approach for satisfactory medical care.[1]

The immediate effects of rationing on the emergency medical system are most evident when time is crucial. It is here that delays and
overloading lead rapidly to breakdowns in the system, which consequently increase mortality and morbidity. When the EMS is over-

whelmed, it becomes dysfunctional, as it has become on many occasions. The results are most evident in the high mortality rates among high-risk patients.

RATIONING OF EMERGENCY MEDICAL SERVICES IN THE INNER CITY

For the 9 million inhabitants of Los Angeles County, which has the largest EMS system in the country, about one-half of the sixteen thousand emergency trauma admissions per year are currently cared for in private hospitals; the other half receive care in Los Angeles County public hospitals. About four thousand trauma admissions are managed by Los Angeles County–USC Medical Center, and approximately the same number are handled at King-Drew Medical Center, located in Watts. Both are inner-city public hospitals; both are patient-taxed to the point of disarray; and the problems are manifold.

Overcrowding occurs during those periods when no beds are available for patients requiring admission, and these patients cannot be accommodated in neighboring facilities.[2] In some large metropolitan areas, patients often wait for days for admission to the emergency department. The syndrome of too many patients requiring acute in-patient care when too few hospital beds are available to accommodate them has become known as "emergency department gridlock."[3]

The gridlock metaphor refers to configurations of interlocking stretchers that now characterize most large inner-city public hospitals, making it difficult to walk from stretcher to stretcher and back to the nurses' station. In California, paramedics and emergency medical technicians cannot unload their patients from their stretchers. This condition immobilizes prehospital care units and thereby renders them incapable of responding efficiently to other patients requiring urgent care.

Because of the aforementioned state of paralysis, many patients in the emergency department's waiting rooms are not seen for prolonged periods, if at all. Hockberger and others observed that when people arrive at the waiting room and realize that they will have to wait between four and eighteen hours before they can see a physician, they will often refuse to register. In a large metropolitan inner-city emergency department, the number of patients who walk away from the waiting room without registering is four to five times greater than the number who register.[4] At King-Drew Medical Center in 1990, 3,014 (8.5 percent) of 35,376 patients left after registering without having been seen by a physician, and about four to five times that number (30 to 40 percent) left without registering, because either the emergency department was closed or the waiting period was too long. This situation clearly demonstrates that when patients finally get into the health care system, it is frequently too late in the course of the disease to salvage either life or limb.

King-Drew Medical Center may, on any occasion, have more than twenty patients who, though "admitted" to the hospital, are still occupying a bed in the emergency department observation area because a hospital bed is not yet available. In these instances, every hospital bed, critical-care-unit bed, and postanesthesia recovery bed are filled, which compels patients to recover in the operating room.

During the past six months at King-Drew, there have been as many as eleven emergency department patients at one time on mechanical ventilation, and patient deaths have resulted from those acute inadequacies. At some point, the hospital shuts down for new admissions, but this often does not prevent paramedics from bringing in additional patients. Moreover, 40 percent of the patients arrive via their own transportation, and it is impossible to prevent their entry, although the hospital may be "officially" closed to ambulances. Moreover, when the other county facilities are also "closed," the center is of necessity "open," despite the inability to provide proper care.

The snowball effect of delays not only increases shock and mortality but also increases the incidence of shock-related multiple organ failures, which can lead to multiple costs before the preventable death. Conjointly, delays tie up scarce and expensive resources and preclude their use for more salvageable patients.

HEALTH INSURANCE COVERAGE FOR VIOLENCE-RELATED TRAUMA

Approximately 40 percent of the U.S. population is either uninsured or underinsured, which creates a burden on the private sector that cannot be met by charity care alone. In Los Angeles, unreimbursed care by private institutions exceeds $3 billion a year. The lack of basic health insurance for all Americans has led to the closing of community hospitals and trauma centers as well as to the downgrading of emergency departments throughout the Los Angeles area. Twenty-one of the original thirty-one private hospitals that initially were committed to the countywide trauma program have withdrawn from the system after less than two years of operation because the small percentage of operating costs that was recovered jeopardized the institutions' solvency. Some of these hospitals reported losses of between $1 million and $2 million annually on their emergency services. Implicit in these changes is the tacit desire to actively prevent, or passively avoid, having uninsured patients enter the private hospital network. Poverty breeds crime, and violence leads to a high incidence of intentional penetrating trauma. People with gunshot wounds and stab wounds, which are penetrating injuries, are rarely covered by insurance. By contrast, people in motor vehicle accidents are usually covered by insurance. This means that suburban community hospitals are well remunerated for trauma, but inner-city public hospitals are not.

If critical-care-unit beds are tied up with victims of violence, the hospital must limit care to less urgent patients. Elective operations and procedures for insured patients, by contrast, are usually reimbursed by third-party payers. Institutions admitting nonpaying trauma patients to the Intensive Care Unit (ICU) may become fiscally unsound. If this goes unchecked, ultimately the hospital may be unable to provide any care to the uninsured. In addition, when a surgical team and the operative capacity of the hospital are involved with penetrating trauma, they are unavailable for other emergencies.

HEALTH CARE AND SOCIAL PATHOLOGIES: A CASE STUDY

It is evident that in the inner city there is filial bond between poverty and violence, which directly affects the health care system. The following case history illustrates with poignancy this "social truth." E. P., a nineteen-year-old black male, entered the emergency room with gunshot wounds to the chest and abdomen. As a result, he sustained injury to diaphragm, liver, stomach, colon, ileum, and spleen. After ten operations and multiple organ failures (including acute respiratory distress syndrome, renal failure, hepatic failure, and sepsis), 157 days in the ICU, and 179 hospital days, the patient died. The hospital costs (not charges) approached a half million dollars. The disturbing fact is that the prevention of the tragedy was possible at three points. Appropriate education and job opportunity could have provided an alternative to the drug economy, which led to the shooting. Then, delays in the young man's initial resuscitation and clinical management contributed to postoperative shock, multiple vital organ failure, hospital costs, and death. Finally, early social and legal intervention would have steered the young man toward a different course.

CONCLUSION

In closing, although much of the talk of rationing has concerned the Oregon proposal and its impact on health care delivery in the near future, rationing is already a fact of life for the millions of poor and either underinsured or uninsured in this country. The lack of comprehensive universal health insurance has led to gross reimbursement inequities, which have resulted in the outright closure of trauma centers and community hospitals. The most profound impact has been in the so-called front end of the health care system—the emergency departments of public hospitals. Those that have not closed have been forced to limit their services or are subject to qualitative rationing, so that the services they do provide are often less than optimal. The ongoing crisis in health care demands a comprehensive approach that addresses our social, as well as medical, ills.

NOTES

1. Richard H. Cales, "Trauma Mortality in Orange County: The Effect of Implementation of a Regional Trauma System," *Annals of Emergency Medicine*, vol. 13 (December 1984), p. 1157; and Steven R. Shackford and others, "Impact of a Trauma System on Outcome of Severely Injured Patients," *Archives of Surgery*, vol. 122 (May 1987), pp. 523–27.

2. Stephan G. Lynn and others, "Critical Decision Making: Managing the Emergency Department in an Overcrowded Hospital," *Annals of Emergency Medicine*, vol. 20 (March 1991), pp. 287–92.

3. Lynn and others, "Critical Decision Making"; and E. J. Gallagher and

others, "The Etiology of Medical Gridlock: Causes of Emergency Department Overcrowding in New York City," *Journal of Emergency Medicine*, vol. 8 (November–December 1990), pp. 785–90.

4. R. S. Hockberger and others, "Hospital Overcrowding: When the Emergency Department Is Open and the Hospital Is Closed," American College of Emergency Physicians, Scientific Assembly, San Francisco, September 16, 1990.

Legal and Philosophical Reflections

E. HAAVI MORREIM

Rationing and the Law

After many years of a health care economy that provided generous reimbursements for providers and ample benefits for patients, an exponential escalation of the cost of care has given rise to major efforts to trim expenditures.[1] The nation's outlays for health care have grown at double-digit levels for many years, and those who pay the bill—government, businesses, insurers, and patients themselves—have instituted assorted devices to contain their costs. The resulting resource constraints pose serious moral and legal challenges for physicians.

Morally, many physicians believe they cannot provide their patients with the level of care they owe if inadequate resources preclude their ordering important diagnostic tests, offering optimal therapies, or hospitalizing patients who need it. The problem is particularly poignant because the people who are most often affected by these shortages are the poor. Thirty-plus million people who have no medical insurance, and indeed many more who have inadequate insurance, often find that their only source of care is a public hospital that is increasingly unable to support its growing population of indigent patients.[2]

Legally, physicians face a vexing jurisprudential dilemma that juxtaposes longstanding legal expectations with new economic realities. Traditionally, law expects all physicians' care to measure up to at least a certain quality—a standard of care. That standard has three features of special interest here.[3] First, it is essentially unitary. With certain exceptions for variations in physicians' training and in geographic availability of resources, malpractice law expects the physician to deliver the same basic quality of care to every patient whom he accepts for care.*

*Throughout this paper I observe the somewhat old-fashioned but still correct custom of using the masculine pronoun in its gender-neutral form to

Second, the standard of care is also largely blind to economics. A physician is usually free to refuse someone as a patient for any reason, including indigency. But once he has accepted a patient for care, he must deliver the same basic quality, regardless of whether the patient can pay. To do less may be regarded as abandonment.

Third, the standard of care has increasingly come to incorporate technologies. Through an assortment of cases, courts have held that physicians must "take X-ray pictures, or have them taken,"[4] order pathological examinations of tissue, perform various tests, and keep patients in hospitals as long as medically necessary.[5]

Courts have placed these duties directly on physicians, with little interest in who owns the technologies or who pays for their use. That indifference was not without warrant, because for many years medical resources were managed in a system amounting to "medical communism." Insured patients were charged in excess of the actual cost of their care, creating extra funds to cover uncompensated care— "from each according to his means, to each according to his needs." Although not everyone had access to the system, those who did could receive a fairly full range of its benefits. In this way, it was fairly easy for physicians to deliver to poorer patients the same basic level of care, including technologies, that they gave to their well-funded patients.

Recently, however, widespread cost containment has turned this traditional equality into an impossible command. Medical communism is disappearing as insurers and businesses are no longer willing to pay for the care of indigents alongside their own beneficiaries. Using special arrangements such as preferred provider organizations, these payers arrange for discounts that cover only the care of their own employees or subscribers, with little or none of the traditional surplus to cover uncompensated care. With these reduced fees, providers such as hospitals and physicians are less able to accept the number of indigent patients they once did. The result is that those uninsured patients are increasingly concentrated in public facilities

---

stand as the singular indefinite pronoun. To use 'they' and 'their' mistakenly places a plural pronoun where there ought to be a singular; consistently using the feminine pronoun instead of the masculine is no less 'biased'; and alternating between the two seems awkward and contrived. Though I use the masculine pronoun, no gender bias is intended.

whose resources are commensurately constrained in caring for their burgeoning numbers. Otherwise stated, the situation is one of "stratified scarcity" in which the level of care available to well-funded patients far exceeds that available to the underinsured and uninsured. It has become impossible, in many instances, to provide these latter patients with the same level of care routinely delivered to the majority.

Despite these profound economic changes, the legal standard of care remains largely unchanged: it requires physicians to deliver a roughly unitary level of care, including important technologies, to all patients, regardless of their ability to pay. Because of this, when economic constraints do not permit the physician to deliver all the care that is otherwise standard, the physician stands to be held personally liable for limitations that are completely beyond his control. If, for example, a crowded public hospital does not have enough beds to hospitalize all patients who need it for as long as they need it, the physician might be held liable for a decision to discharge a patient prematurely, even though fairness to other needier patients, or a sheer lack of beds, might have necessitated the discharge.[6]

Two answers to this jurisprudential problem are most commonly offered. If there is a clash between resource stratification and the unitary standard of care, one option is to keep the standard of care unitary as it now is, despite resource inequalities, in hopes of pressuring physicians to make the best possible use of available resources.[7] Alternatively, resources could be equalized, thus eliminating the conflict between legal standards and economic realities.

In the first answer, scholars argue that there is really very little problem in the first place. The law permits physicians to streamline and vary the standard of care to some degree. If physicians stretch resources further, they can largely mitigate the problem.[8] If genuine rationing must occur one day, society as a whole should make such decisions, and should adjust the standard of care accordingly. Meanwhile, physicians must hold fast to their ethic of patient advocacy.[9]

This first resolution is problematic. It essentially denies that stratified scarcity really exists: if only we are a bit more frugal, we can make the problem go away. And yet, ample evidence is emerging to document that those who care for the poor now are often unable, regardless of their frugality, to deliver the care that is standard elsewhere in the health care system.[10]

It is also problematic because it presumes that physicians retain a control over resources that they have actually lost. Physicians no longer command resources with just a signature, as they once did. Hospitals, insurers, and others who own or pay for the tools that physicians use have installed a formidable array of controls. Some limit physicians' decisions directly, as when a hospital's pharmacy does not stock certain costly drugs. Incentives influence physicians indirectly through a system of bonuses and penalties. The physician can pay a substantial personal price if his decisions are not sufficiently cost-conscious or profit-producing.[11] No matter how dedicated to serving the patient, the physician cannot single-handedly remove the powerful economic constraints that now limit his actions.

Even more important, it seems morally untenable to suppose that physicians can owe what they neither own nor control. Admittedly, the U.S. health care system has long empowered physicians to use whatever resources they wish in the care of their patients. Indeed, until recently, a retrospective, fee-for-service reimbursement system encouraged health care providers to do as much as possible, as expensively as possible, for every patient. And yet, when viewed objectively instead of historically, that sort of arrangement appears quite extraordinary.

It is extraordinary, for example, to presume that physicians are morally entitled to dictate how much money others must spend for a patient's care, solely because they have judged that the patient needs it. Surely there is something both morally and practically odd about a society that requires physicians virtually to commandeer others' money and property without being concerned about how much of whose resources they take. Reciprocally, it is at least as odd that this system threatens to penalize physicians substantially should they fail to conscript the expected level of resources, despite the fact that those who own these resources have now asserted strong controls over them.[12]

The second resolution above would have us equalize resources.[13] Equality, however, can be attained in only two ways: either enough money must be spent to provide every citizen every intervention that the currently rather lavish standard of care now embraces, or everyone must be coerced to accept the considerably more modest standard that could be realistically afforded for all citizens.[14] The former option would be exorbitantly costly, while the latter unduly restricts individuals' freedom to spend their money as they wish, including to purchase health care. As Blumstein and Sloan have suggested, a literal equality of resources may be both unattainable and undesirable.

> Leveling up would require such a staggering commitment of resources that other public priorities would unduly suffer; leveling down would promote gross inefficiency, lower quality, achieve a dubious sort of equity in which waiting time would be the main resource allocator, and threaten fundamental precepts of freedom by barring individual expenditures for health above some arbitrary limit set by government.[15]

THE DIVIDED STANDARD OF CARE: RATIONALE

These first two answers, then, must be rejected. It is a mistake to ignore the very real inequality of resources, and equally wrong to presume that physicians can and should be the principal arbiters of resource allocation. An entirely different approach is needed to our jurisprudential dilemma. Somehow a distinction must be made between what physicians are expected to do for their patients and the ways in which resources are allocated. Accordingly, instead of speaking about *the* standard of care—a single, comprehensive standard owed exclusively by physicians and encompassing everything from physicians' professional skills to costly technologies—a distinction must be made between that which physicians owe their patients, and the monetary and technological resources that insurers and others may owe a patient. The standard of care must accordingly be divided into two elements: the standard of medical expertise (SME) and the standard of resource use (SRU).

The SME, as I propose it, is the standard to which we would hold the physician accountable. It is the level of knowledge, skill, and effort that he is expected to deliver to every patient whom he accepts for care, regardless of the patient's income. The surgeon has no right to make careless incisions, nor the internist to make hasty diagnostic inferences, just because the patient is poor. The SME does, however, have a resource component. Although no one would expect the physician to commandeer others' resources on his patients' behalf, or to "game the system" to trick insurers into paying for care that they would not otherwise cover, one would expect physicians to be vigorous economic advocates for their patients.[16] That advocacy would include helping the patient to meet utilization review requirements, for instance, or to help with claim forms necessary for insurance reimbursement.[17]

The SRU, as I define it, is the level of medical and monetary resources to which the patient is legally entitled.[18] Physicians must, of course, have some role in identifying the kind of care that is most suitable for a given condition and thereby in defining what level of resources ought, ideally, to be provided. But the actual level of resources to which a given patient is legally entitled is a function, not of what some physician thinks he needs, but of what care or coverage the patient or others have purchased for him. That entitlement may be a comprehensive policy with "first dollar" coverage for all needed care, or a minimal coverage provided under a state medicaid plan, or it may be nothing more than the emergency care that a hospital with an emergency department must provide for anyone who comes to its doors.

If a patient has not received a needed resource, the problem might be a breach of the SME or the SRU, or both. If the physician simply did not know that a particular test was indicated, for instance, then there may be an SME failure of medical expertise. Or if he failed to make a required phone call to the patient's insurer for utilization review approval, the problem may be a failure of physician advocacy.[19] If, however, the physician exercised reasonable judgment, skill, and effort, and the failure instead was an insurer's refusal to pay for care that was clearly covered, then the standard that was violated was not the SME but the SRU.[20]

The divided standard of care might appear to be a rather novel idea. After all, the standard of care in malpractice law has always been something that the physician alone owes each patient, and it has always been owed to each patient equally. Here I propose that physicians do not owe others' resources to their patients, and that those who do owe resources do not owe them in equal measure to every patient. That is, I propose a "divided standard of care" with a "variable SRU."

On closer examination, this approach is actually not so novel. Current practices and many existing legal doctrines actually support a divided standard of care, including an SRU that can vary from patient to patient. What may seem novel is actually what we (nearly) already do.

THE DIVIDED STANDARD OF CARE: LEGAL SUPPORT

Earlier I argued that it makes rational and moral sense for malpractice law to distinguish between a standard of medical expertise and a standard of resource use, and to acknowledge that medical resources— the SRU—need not be equal for everyone. It is quite another thing to show that this approach is acceptable within the broader scheme of the American legal system. In fact, however, existing statutes and case law already implicitly support the idea of treating resource issues separately from expertise questions. Further, current law permits and even creates wide variations in the health care packages from which people derive their legal entitlement to health care resources (SRUs). Later I will explain how medical mishaps could be litigated under a divided standard of care, and I will show how a divided standard of care can offer patients as good or better legal protection from medical mishaps than the traditional unitary standard of care.

Variable SRU

As a matter of economic policy, the government has long permitted a wide variety of health care plans and has itself contributed to that diversity. Federal medicare for the elderly tends to provide considerably better coverage than state medicaid programs for the poor, for example, and states vary widely in their eligibility requirements and benefit packages for medicaid.[21]

Such variation is entirely permissible under law. First, states are not obligated to participate in the medicaid program or to provide health care benefits at all to their citizens. "The constitution imposes no obligation on the States . . . to pay any of the medical expenses of indigents."[22] Second, although those that do participate must cover certain categories of services such as inpatient hospital services and physicians' services, they need not provide funding for all varieties of treatment within those categories.[23] Further, states are free to alter, and even to reduce, their benefits packages. "The benefit provided through Medicaid is a particular package of health care services, such as 14 days of inpatient coverage. That package of services has the general aim of assuring that individuals will receive necessary medical care, but the benefit provided remains the individual services offered—not 'adequate health care.'"[24]

Thus, people with different kinds of government health care insurance can have very different resource entitlements. Businesses often provide considerably more lavish benefits packages for their employees than governments do for their beneficiaries, yet even within this realm there is considerable diversity. Although many states mandate that certain benefits be provided in any health insurance policy, many states expressly waive these requirements for small businesses, to enable them to purchase at least a minimum health package for their employees rather than none at all.[25] In the same vein, Congress's Pepper Commission explicitly recommended that mandated benefits be waived to enable small companies to furnish insurance for their employees.[26] Under these rules, one finds explicit legal acceptance of the notion that employees of small firms might be entitled to a lesser SRU than those working for major corporations.

Even well-funded insurance programs differ widely. Of particular interest, many third-party payers assemble their own guidelines by which to decide for which interventions they will pay. In most cases these guidelines are detailed criteria whereby a utilization reviewer determines whether a particular intervention is medically necessary and, thereby, reimbursable. It is the insurer's own medical necessity standard, and because insurers generally do not share these "cookbooks" with subscribers, providers, or one another, they vary considerably. Health Maintenance Organizations (HMOs), similarly, have their own criteria defining the standard health care they provide for their subscribers. Again, there is nothing illegal about these sometimes highly idiosyncratic guidelines, nor in the wide variations among them.

Divided Standard of Care

Aside from this explicit legal permission for wide variations among resource packages, several legal doctrines support the notion that even the traditional unitary standard of care can be altered in light of

resource constraints. In this sense, current law acknowledges that resource problems are somehow different from professional expertise.

The locality rule, for example, has long permitted a lower standard
of care in remote rural areas. In the 1800s, when the locality rule was
created, physicians in remote areas were unable to gain access to the
latest medical information or to hone their skills as regularly as physicians in highly populated areas. Fairness dictated that they not be
held to a standard they could not achieve.[27] In the present era of in-
stant communication and standardized medical training, courts have
rightly discarded locality as an excuse for ignorance or carelessness.[28]
However, the locality rule has been revised and retained to encom-
pass resource constraints. Many rural areas do not have the sophisticated technologies that are available in the cities, and the same concept of fairness dictates that these differences be acknowledged.[29] In
this sense, the locality rule has been discarded as a way of altering the
SME, but retained to vary the SRU.

In addition, the traditional standard of care has never required an
ossification of existing practices. Courts can permit physicians' customs to evolve over time. And to allow for change and improvement
and for legitimate differences of opinion within the profession, courts
have accepted the noncustomary practices of reputable minorities. In
this way, courts can accept considerable economizing of medical practices, so long as they preserve basic quality of care.[30]

Also relevant are those cases and doctrines that expressly permit
physicians and hospitals to enjoy reduced liability for negligence in
their care of the poor. The doctrine of charitable immunity has long
permitted charitable hospitals either to be exempt from liability for
negligence or to bear only a low, strictly fixed limit of liability. Initially,
the doctrine emerged to ensure that costly litigation would not deter
potential contributors from their generosity, but over the years it was
nearly abandoned on the ground that hospitals "should be just before
they are generous."[31] In recent years, however, it has been reinvigo-
rated. Arguing that charitable hospitals' limited resources might be
better spent on patient care than on malpractice premiums, a number
of courts have recently held that such liability limits do not violate
either equal protection or due process and that they serve the legitimate state interest of keeping charity care available for the poor.[32]

In a similar vein, some states have expressly given immunity to
physicians who care for the indigent. Tennessee, for example, en-

acted a Community Health Agency Act in 1989 to encourage physicians to care for uninsured patients by encompassing such care within the liability protections of the state's sovereign immunity. Under that immunity, damages for any malpractice claims are restricted to $300,000 per claimant and $1,000,000 per occurrence.[33] Similarly, an Illinois law provides that physicians who care for patients at established free clinics, and who do not accept any remuneration for such care, are immune from civil liability so long as they are acting in good faith and do not engage in wanton or willful misconduct.[34]

It should be mentioned that these charitable and sovereign immunities do not literally permit physicians and hospitals to practice poorer care or to deliver a lesser level of resources. Rather, they limit the patient's recovery in the event of negligent or inadequate care.[35] Still, from the patient's point of view, the effect is essentially the same. Because the patient has lesser entitlement to recovery for injuries resulting from substandard care, he has, in effect, lesser entitlement to standard care in the first place.[36] In the process, the law has distinguished on economic grounds what providers owe to their poorer patients.

The clearest case of a divided standard of care comes from Oregon. In 1989 its legislature created a priority-based resource system that explicitly recognizes that its medicaid recipients may have a lesser SRU than privately insured citizens typically receive. The statute requires that various medical services be ranked in order of importance, and from there the level of resources that beneficiaries receive can vary from year to year, depending on the state budget. A higher allocation means that more services on the priority list will be funded, while in a lean year medicaid recipients will be entitled to fewer services. Because the state is attempting to provide health care for many more citizens with roughly the same amount of money, it is likely that current beneficiaries will receive fewer services when the plan is implemented than they do now.[37]

Interestingly, the Oregon legislature has already anticipated and responded to the jurisprudential challenge addressed in this paper. Recognizing the potentially disastrous malpractice implications for physicians who might be forced to deny medicaid patients care that would ordinarily be considered standard, the state has granted sweeping immunity for physicians when their care of these patients is curtailed by the state's priority-based funding decisions. In effect, then, the state has explicitly acknowledged that its own legislature, not the physician, is responsible for the standard of resource use that medicaid patients are to receive. In so doing, Oregon expressly divides the standard of care: "Any health care provider or plan contracting to provide services to the eligible population . . . shall not be subject to criminal prosecution, civil liability or professional disciplinary action for failing to provide a service which the Legislative Assembly has not funded or has eliminated from its funding pursuant to ORS 414.735."[38]

In sum, there is considerable evidence to show that the U.S. legal system can embrace a divided standard of care that distinguishes between the SME and the SRU and that permits a variable SRU rather than requiring a unitary level of resources for all patients. It is another matter, however, to demonstrate that patients could enjoy adequate legal protection against medical mishaps under such a system.

LITIGATION UNDER THE DIVIDED STANDARD OF CARE

To discuss what remedies patients would have under the divided standard of care, one must consider the SME and the SRU separately. The former is most suitably managed in tort; the latter in contract. Tort law concerns the general conduct that people expect of one another. One does not expect perfection, but people should treat one another with a reasonable amount of care, so as to avoid causing harm. In recent years, tort has become the primary locus for resolving personal injury cases, including medical malpractice.

Contract differs from tort in that the parties themselves specify what sort of conduct they expect of one another. Where tort imposes upon everyone an expectation to behave as a reasonable and prudent person (or, in the case of medicine, as a reasonable and prudent physician), contractors can decide for themselves who will be expected to do what, and what measures will be taken if one of them fails to fulfill his end of the agreement. In health care, for example, there are contracts between patients and insurers that specify what premium the subscriber will pay in exchange for how much reimbursement of which health care services.

Litigating the SME

The standard of medical expertise is the knowledge, skill, and effort that the physician owes his patient. This standard retains many of the ideals embedded in the traditional standard of care—quality, equality, and a blindness to resource constraints. The physician must deliver the same level of professional expertise to every patient whom he accepts for care, regardless of whether that patient can pay. Because he is free to reject the indigent at the outset, he cannot later cite the patient's inability to pay to excuse carelessness or ignorance.

Further, this expertise is established on a national, not locality-specific, basis. Although one can still differentiate between the level of skill and knowledge to be expected for different subspecialties, one can embrace a truly national SME for physicians within any particular specialty.[39]

Also consistent with the traditional standard of care, the SME should be established by the medical profession. Few outsiders have the expertise to determine what constitutes adequate professional judgment and performance. Likewise, the most plausible way to define the content of the SME is to look to the prevailing customs of the profession, following current practice, with reasonable exceptions made for reputable minorities.

Finally, and again consistent with the traditional standard of care, litigation under the SME would ordinarily be handled within tort law. Although the physician-patient relationship usually begins with an implicit, if not explicit, contract, personal injuries that occur because of negligent medical care are usually regarded as matters of tort. Tort, with its better compensation for personal injuries and its unitary standard of care, often has greater protection for patients.

It should be noted that some scholars favor contractual remedies for malpractice, including for the SME. A patient wanting to reduce the costs of malpractice coverage and thereby to reduce the physician's fees, for example, might agree to submit all claims to arbitration, to accept caps on damages, or perhaps even to embrace a no-fault approach.[40] However, even if one agrees that physicians and patients ought to have some freedom to arrange their own liability standards, there are reasons to be cautious. Courts have shied away from contracts in which the patient must grant the provider complete exculpation for negligence, arguing that an ill patient seeking medical help is placed in an impossible position when asked to sign such a contract as a prerequisite for care. The patient is usually in a much weaker bargaining position and has few, if any, alternatives to signing. Therefore, the courts have ruled, such exculpatory clauses are not binding.[41] Not all contracting over the SME would necessarily embrace an exculpatory clause, of course, but these cases do indicate that tort remains the preferred avenue for litigating the SME and that any contractual alteration would have to include extensive protections for patients.

Litigating the SRU

In discussing patients' legal recourse for inappropriate resource decisions, one must distinguish between those instances in which the patient is privately insured and those in which he is funded by the government.

PRIVATE INSURANCE. To argue that patients' resource entitlements should be managed under contract rather than tort is hardly revolutionary. The economic aspects of health care are traditionally managed under contract law. When physicians try to collect unpaid bills from patients, they do so under contract law. Similarly, medical insurance law is a matter of contract. As with every other kind of insurance, a person pays a premium in exchange for a specified, limited list of benefits. If either party reneges on his part of the bargain, the other can sue him to make it right.

Under a divided standard of care, a patient is not entitled to receive whatever level of resources a physician thinks he needs, or whatever level physicians customarily order for their patients. Rather, the patient is legally entitled to whatever resources he bought, or are furnished for him by third parties such as an employer or government. In this sense, the SRU enforced for any particular person is the one that he himself has chosen, or that he has voluntarily accepted from someone else. Although the current system that leaves so many citizens without any legal entitlement to health care might be vigorously challenged on moral, economic, and practical grounds, it can also be acknowledged that when there are clear agreements, it is reasonable to address them under contract law.[42]

This means that if a person has voluntarily and knowledgeably purchased an insurance policy, he should ordinarily be bound by the terms of that policy. Case precedent supports this stance. Where an insurance policy provides that an insurer may retrospectively deny payment for care that is not medically necessary, for example, courts have upheld the insurer's right to enforce this provision—even though that may sometimes mean that the subscriber finds himself unexpectedly without coverage for an intervention that his physician told him was necessary.[43]

Aside from the traditional management of health insurance under contract law, one could cite other legal doctrines that can require people to abide by the SRUs they have chosen. One potentially relevant doctrine is "assumption of risk." When a person enters into an activity acknowledging and freely assuming its risks, he exonerates in advance those who might otherwise be liable for the creation of those risks.[44] In the case of *Schneider* v. *Revici*, a woman who was diagnosed as having breast cancer rejected surgery and radiation in favor of unconventional nutrition therapy. The physician providing that alternative care clearly informed her that the therapy was not approved and also, once it had clearly proved ineffective for her, advised her several times to seek conventional treatment. When the woman finally did consult a surgeon, her disease had progressed too far for hope of cure. She sued the first physician over his worthless remedies, and the court held that, in agreeing to opt for unapproved therapy despite its clearly stated risks, she had assumed the risk and could not hold the physician liable for her own choice.[45]

If applied to patients' insurance choices, the doctrine of assumption of risk could help courts to acknowledge that when a person has knowingly chosen an insurance package that excludes certain coverages, he has expressly assumed a risk: namely, the risk that he might incur the very health problem whose coverage he rejected.[46] Although such choices have their hazards, they nevertheless are consistent with the autonomy that we insist upon elsewhere in our lives—such as the freedom to purchase a less crashworthy automobile and thereby to incur a greater risk of bodily harm.[47]

It may also be noted that litigating the SRU under contract, as described here, does not fall prey to some of the traditional arguments against using contract to resolve questions about the SME standard of care. As mentioned, courts have steadfastly rejected contracts with exculpatory clauses freeing physicians from liability for negligence.[48]

An ill patient might "agree" to exonerate the physician for negligence as a condition for receiving care, but his choice was hardly free if he was in urgent need of medical intervention and unable to seek help elsewhere. In this sense, one might discourage contracting over the SME.

Contracting for the SRU, however, is entirely different. A person selecting a health insurance plan is ordinarily not ill nor is his competence impaired. He is quite as able to evaluate information about these choices as he is about many other choices, so long as he is presented with ample, good-quality information. When large groups of patients or large employers can bargain on roughly equal terms with insurers, patients may be even less vulnerable to being treated unfairly in negotiations.[49] Similarly, when patients are presented with a number of different options, they can exercise their own power of the purse by opting for those plans that provide the best benefits at the best cost. Thus, it is consistent with longstanding legal traditions to litigate the SRU in contract, including to hold patients to the contracts by which they establish their own SRU.

Although the law permits people to contract for health insurance and generally expects them to abide by the terms of their agreements, it also provides considerable protection for patients, in light of their special vulnerabilities in this particular contractual setting.[50] First, courts can be harsh with insurers that attempt to cheat patients or to interfere inappropriately with delivery of care. A recent California case, for instance, opened the door to negligence suits against third-party payers whose utilization review or other cost containment programs result in medically inappropriate decisions. If arbitrary denial of payment results in a premature discharge of a patient from the hospital and thereby leads to patient injury, for instance, the third-party payer might be liable for negligence.[51] It will be important for courts to distinguish carefully between those cases in which an insurer denies a benefit in accordance with the subscriber's policy and those in which it carelessly or perniciously deprives the patient of benefits to which he is entitled. Only in the latter kind of case should the patient's injuries be legitimately ascribed to an insurer.

Second, in keeping with the general principle that contracts are to be construed against their drafters, insurance law usually favors the insured. Ambiguities in policies are interpreted in the subscriber's favor, and any exceptions or limits on coverage must be specified in clear language.[52] Thus, when there is a question about whether the subscriber was entitled to a particular benefit, the court is likely to rule that he was.

Beyond this, insurance contracts commonly receive close scrutiny by courts because they are typically contracts of adhesion in which the purchaser has no opportunity to negotiate the terms of the agreement or to alter the policy to suit his preferences. One can only "take it or leave it," and because ordinarily one has substantial need for the service in question, "leaving it" is usually not a viable option.[53]

Fiduciary law provides further protection. Insurers are sometimes regarded as fiduciaries because they have vastly greater power than their subscribers. When such a relationship exists, the fiduciary (insurer) is expected to give beneficiaries complete and candid information and to consider the beneficiary's interests at least as highly as its own. [54]

In some instances an even more powerful kind of lawsuit is available. If an insurer has egregiously failed to behave in good faith, as when it deliberately and maliciously deprives a subscriber of benefits it clearly owes, the patient may be able to bring suit under the doctrine of "bad faith breach of contract." Such suits can be lodged in either tort or contract, but are most commonly brought under tort law, because judgments there can include punitive and noneconomic as well as economic damages.[55]

Breach of warranty is yet another potential basis for suit. If an insurer or HMO advertises that it provides only the best and most complete care, but then fails to disclose major limits on coverage, there may be a breach of warranty. The same scenario might also give rise to a case for fraud or misrepresentation.[56]

Finally, some states have specific statutes requiring insurers to conduct their utilization review within specified guidelines, or at least to report regularly on their review staff and activities. Such requirements, if violated, could present further grounds on which an aggrieved patient could sue for relief.[57]

GOVERNMENT INSURANCE. The SRU provided through government insurance might be challenged on two levels. First, one could argue that the government ought to provide more than it does—that it ought to ensure some adequate level of care for all citizens, for instance, or that the benefits it does provide ought to be greater. Second, one could argue that the government ought to keep its commitments better and fully provide the benefits that are already promised in its programs.

Those seeking better government health programs probably cannot hope to achieve them through litigation. There is no constitutional right to health care, nor must existing government health insurance include comprehensive benefits.[58] Legislation, not litigation, is the only real hope for changing government programs.

If there is little ground on which to demand better benefits or wider eligibility, however, there is precedent to require government to deliver fully what it has promised both to patients and to providers. In one recent case, the Virginia Hospital Association sued the Commonwealth of Virginia on the grounds that medicaid payments to providers in that state were not "reasonable and adequate," as required by the Boren amendment to the medicaid legislation. The United States Supreme Court held that providers—particularly hospitals and nursing care facilities—have an enforceable right to adequate compensation for services provided in efficiently and economically run facilities.[59]

Another case concerns the level of care actually provided. A citizens' council in Washington, D.C., successfully sought injunctive and declaratory relief to require improvements at D.C. General Hospital. The group alleged major and ongoing problems in eight areas of the hospital, including its emergency room, medical records, radiology department, and several other services. The circuit court found that the hospital's care fell "well below any acceptable level of quality and efficiency,"[60] and that it had thereby seriously failed to fulfill its legal mandate to deliver "comprehensive hospital care and treatment."[61] Accordingly, the court required the District of Columbia to fill all budgeted positions and to submit a detailed plan of further corrective action.[62]

It is important to note that such avenues of recourse are limited. In some cases, courts have held that even where government has a duty to provide health care to its citizens, that duty must be read in light of competing responsibilities. In 1970 the city of Philadelphia, for example, instituted a hiring freeze that led to understaffing and seriously compromised quality of care at Philadelphia General Hospital— the only source of health care available for many indigent Philadelphians. On appeal, the commonwealth court dismissed the issue as moot because the hiring freeze had been lifted. In its dicta, however, the court held that assuming the correctness of appellants' contention that indigent persons are legally entitled to minimally adequate hospital care provided by the city, the extent of the city's duty would depend upon all the circumstances existing at a given time, including other similarly mandated public needs and the public means. Conceivably, there could be a judicial determination that the performance of the duty might be declared to have been inadequate, adequate, or properly temporarily suspended or contracted based upon circumstances then existent.[63]

In 1976, when the city wanted to close down the hospital entirely, a commonwealth court ruled that the city was entitled to do so, despite its adverse impact on indigent citizens in the city.[64]

Together, these cases tell us that patients insured by the government have few rights to demand more or better health care programs. A government need not promise to deliver the same level of care that is standard for the well-funded majority of citizens, and it can change and even diminish those promises.[65] In other words, government can provide a distinctly lower SRU than that which better-funded citizens enjoy. However, patients and providers do have at least some standing to insist that the government deliver what it has promised.

CONCLUSION

It is striking to note how closely the Oregon Plan fits with the divided standard of care and variable SRU, as recommended here. While expanding access to near-universal levels, its priority-based allocation plan openly establishes a specific, and rather modest, SRU for medicaid recipients. They will receive whatever care lies above the funding line, but are not assured of anything below it. That entitlement can change from year to year as the legislature determines how richly it will fund medicaid. Further, the plan acknowledges publicly that its level of resources may differ from that routinely delivered to well-insured patients, and recognizes that physicians should not be held legally liable for resource inadequacies caused by the state. As noted earlier, physicians are therefore granted explicit immunity where they are unable to deliver resources that would otherwise be considered standard.

Through these provisions, the Oregon Plan becomes the first public experiment in implementing a divided standard of care with a variable SRU. Several conditions are needed to maximize its chances for success. First, the SRU that it establishes each year must be as clear as possible. It is probably not enough simply to say, for example, that the treatment of bacterial meningitis and other specified ailments will be covered. The state must aggressively conduct technology assessment and must create fairly specific guidelines to indicate what treatments, in particular, are warranted for the medical illnesses and conditions specified on its priority list.[66] Only then can its rationing plan—its promised SRU—be fiscally realistic enough for the state actually to deliver what it has promised. Finally, the state must also keep its promise to physicians. When a medicaid patient's poor outcome can be traced to the lack of a resource that was not covered under that year's SRU, the physician must not be held liable for failing to deliver care that was not his to give.

In the final analysis, it will be necessary to do more than divide the standard of care. Some coherence must be brought to the wildly divergent demands of law, medicine, ethics, and economics. On one level, we might feel that everyone is morally entitled to some basic level of care. But such sentiments are not, at this time, matched by economic or legal entitlements. This chapter has presented the argument that, as a first step, it will be necessary for the legal system to recognize that physicians neither can nor should control others' resources, and to admit that it is acceptable for citizens' resource entitlements to vary. This nation, however, must ensure that all citizens have some reasonable, even if unequal, access to health care resources. Until then, it is profoundly distasteful, even if legally correct, to admit that some citizens have little or no standard of resource use.

NOTES

1. Much of the information in this introductory section can be found, in fuller exposition, in two other articles of mine: E. Haavi Morreim, "Cost Containment and the Standard of Medical Care," *California Law Review*, vol. 75 (October 1987), pp. 1719–63; and "Stratified Scarcity: Redefining the Standard of Care," *Law, Medicine and Health Care*, vol. 17 (Winter 1989), pp. 356–67. In both works, the reader may find extensive further references to other works that discuss malpractice and the standard of care.

2. Jack Hadley, Earl P. Steinberg, and Judith Feder, "Comparison of Uninsured and Privately Insured Hospital Patients: Condition on Admission, Resource Use, and Outcome," *Journal of the American Medical Association*, vol. 265 (January 16, 1991), pp. 374–79; and Andrew B. Bindman, Dennis Keane, and Nicole Lurie, "A Public Hospital Closes: Impact on Patients' Access to Health Care and Health Status," *Journal of the American Medical Association*, vol. 264 (December 12, 1990), pp. 2899–2904.

3. The standard of care is one of four elements that a plaintiff (patient) must prove against the defendant (physician) in a malpractice suit: (1) that the physician owed the patient a duty (standard) of care; (2) that the physician breached this duty; (3) that the patient was injured; and (4) that the breach of duty caused the injury.

4. *Peterson v. Hunt*, 84 P.2d 999 at 1000 (Wash. 1938).

5. *Smith v. Yohe*, 194 A.2d 167 (Pa. 1963); *Wilkinson v. Vesey*, 295 A.2d 676 (R.I. 1972); *Hicks v. United States*, 368 F.2d 626 (1966); *Price v. Neyland*, 320 F.2d 674 (D.C. 1963); *Kingston v. McGrath*, 232 F.2d 495 (Idaho 1956); *Wickline v. State of California*, 228 Cal. Rptr. 661 (Cal. App. 2 Dist. 1986). This is not to say that physicians are required to deliver all technologies the patient needs. There is no precedent, for example, to suggest that the physician must purchase prescription medications out of his own pocket for his poorer patients. Still, a long line of precedents clearly expects physicians to deliver many technologies as part of the standard of care.

6. In *Wickline v. State of California*, 228 Cal. Rptr., a California court of appeals stated, in dicta, that the physician is responsible for the decision to discharge a patient, regardless of financial pressure.

7. Barry R. Furrow, "Medical Malpractice and Cost Containment: Tightening the Screws," *Case Western Reserve Law Review*, vol. 36, no. 4 (1985–86), pp. 985–1032.

8. Law can acknowledge economics through such doctrines as the "locality rule" (which accepts resource variations, for example, between urban and rural areas) and the "respectable minority rule" (which permits physicians to practice differently, that is, more economically, than their colleagues). See Mark A. Hall, "The Malpractice Standard under Health Care Cost Containment," *Law, Medicine and Health Care*, vol. 17 (Winter 1989), pp. 347–55.

9. Edward B. Hirshfeld, "Tort Considerations for Third Party Payors," in Kirk B. Johnson and others, eds., *Legal Implications of Practice Parameters* (Chicago: American Medical Association, 1990), pp. 55–90; and Edward B. Hirshfeld, "Economic Considerations in Treatment Decisions and the Standard of Care in Malpractice Litigation," *Journal of the American Medical Association*, vol. 264 (October 17, 1990), pp. 2004–12.

10. Emily Friedman, "The Uninsured: From Dilemma to Crisis," *Journal of the American Medical Association*, vol. 265 (May 15, 1991), p. 2493; and Hadley,

Steinberg, and Feder, "Comparison of Uninsured and Privately Insured Hospital Patients," pp. 374–79.

11. E. Haavi Morreim, "Fiscal Scarcity and the Inevitability of Bedside Budget Balancing," *Archives of Internal Medicine,* vol. 149 (May 1989), pp. 1012–15; and E. Haavi Morreim, "Cost Containment: Challenging Fidelity and Justice," *Hastings Center Report,* vol. 18 (December 1988), pp. 20–25.

12. E. Haavi Morreim, "Gaming the System: Dodging the Rules, Ruling the Dodgers," *Archives of Internal Medicine,* vol. 151 (March 1991), pp. 443–47.

13. These two approaches—to keep the standard of care unitary despite resource inequalities or to render resources equal—are not the only two that have been offered in response to this jurisprudential problem. Some observers have proposed that special exceptions should be made for physicians whose care was limited by severe economic constraints (see E. Haavi Morreim, "Cost Containment and the Standard of Medical Care"), while elsewhere there is some sympathy for permitting physicians to allocate resources as they see fit, with relatively little supervision from tort law (see J. A. Siliciano, "Wealth, Equity and the Unitary Medical Malpractice Standard," *Virginia Law Review,* vol. 77 [1991], pp. 439–87).

14. Indeed, Canada has embraced this latter approach, since it forbids private insurance for any care that is covered under its health care system. John K. Iglehart, "Canada's Health Care System Faces Its Problems," *New England Journal of Medicine,* vol. 322 (February 22, 1990), pp. 562–68.

15. James F. Blumstein and Frank A. Sloan, "Redefining Government's Role in Health Care: Is a Dose of Competition What the Doctor Should Order?" *Vanderbilt Law Review,* vol. 34 (May 1981), p. 865.

16. Morreim, "Gaming the System."

17. For a more detailed discussion of what is, and is not, required by economic advocacy, see E. Haavi Morreim, "Economic Disclosure and Economic Advocacy: New Duties in the Medical Standard of Care," *Journal of Legal Medicine,* vol. 12 (September 1991), pp. 275–329.

18. Although one might want to argue that everyone in the nation is morally entitled to receive a basic minimum of care, this article is restricted to law and to current conditions. Under current conditions, many people have no legal entitlement to health care except for certain emergency services.

19. *Wickline* v. *State of California,* 228 Cal. Rptr.; and Morreim, "Economic Disclosure and Economic Advocacy."

20. Gerald W. Grumet, "Health Care Rationing through Inconvenience: The Third Party's Secret Weapon," *New England Journal of Medicine,* vol. 321 (August 31, 1989), pp. 607–11.

21. Friedman, "The Uninsured," p. 2492; and Eli Ginzberg and Miriam Ostow, "Beyond Universal Health Insurance to Effective Health Care," *Journal of the American Medical Association,* vol. 265 (May 15, 1991), pp. 2559–60.

22. *Maher* v. *Roe*, 432 U.S. 464 at 469 (D.C. 1977).

23. *Harris* v. *McRae*, 448 U.S. 297 at 301 (1980).

24. *Alexander* v. *Choate*, 105 S. Ct. 712 at 722 (Tenn. 1985).

25. Hilary Stout, "Insurance Firms Are Criticized on Health Plans," *Wall Street Journal*, June 4, 1991, p. B8.

26. John D. Rockefeller, "The Pepper Commission Report on Comprehensive Health Care," *New England Journal of Medicine*, vol. 323 (October 4, 1990), pp. 1005–07; and P. Wade, "Health Plans Want Small Firms Excluded," *Commercial Appeal*, December 13, 1990, p. B4.

27. *Small* v. *Howard*, 128 Mass. 131 (1880); and *Tefft* v. *Wilcox*, 6 Kan. 46 (1870).

28. *Shilkret* v. *Annapolis Emergency Hospital Ass'n*, 349 A.2d 245 (Md. 1985); and *Brune* v. *Belinkoff*, 235 N.E. 2d 793 (Mass. 1968).

29. *Hall* v. *Hilbun*, 466 So. 2d 856 (Miss. 1985); Morreim, "Cost Containment and the Standard of Medical Care"; and Hall, "The Malpractice Standard under Health Care Cost Containment."

30. Furrow, "Medical Malpractice and Cost Containment"; Morreim, "Cost Containment and the Standard of Medical Care"; and Hall, "Malpractice Standard under Health Care Cost Containment."

31. *Bing* v. *Thiung*, 143 N.E. 2d 3 at 8 (N.Y. 1957).

32. *English* v. *New England Medical Center*, 541 N.E. 2d 329 (Mass. 1989); and *Cutts* v. *Fulton-DeKalb Hospital Authority*, 385 S.E.2d 436 (Ga. App. 1989).

33. Tenn. Code Ann. 68-2-1115; and Tenn. Code Ann. 9-8-307 (3) (e).

34. Ill. Rev. Stat. Ch. 111, sec. 4400–31 (1989).

35. As Robert Baker points out, these uses of charitable and sovereign immunity offer a third standard of care—a standard of restitution—that says the poor may be less entitled to the same restitution for their injuries.

36. In somewhat the same vein, the U.S. government granted civil immunity to physicians who followed guidelines created under the auspices of its Professional Standards Review Organizations (PSROs) in the early 1970s. In a move to promote efficiency, PSROs were charged with creating norms of care for various health conditions—rather like today's "practice parameters." See H. David Banta and Stephen B. Thacker, "The Case for Reassessment of Health Care Technology: Once Is Not Enough," *Journal of the American Medical Association*, vol. 264 (July 11, 1990), pp. 235–240; and Steven H. Woolf, "Practice Guidelines: A New Reality in Medicine," *Archives of Internal Medicine*, vol. 150 (1990), pp. 1811–18. Those guidelines were intended to represent a cost-conscious minimum level of care, and a physician following them could not be held liable for adverse outcomes. See Morreim, "Cost Containment and the Standard of Medical Care," p. 1751. Though PSROs no longer exist, Peer Review Organizations (PROs) were created in 1982 to serve many of the same functions. PROs were not originally charged specifically to develop specific

guidelines, but they do review physicians' care to determine whether payment should be made or withheld and are obligated to establish criteria to guide that review. Any physician whose care comports with those guidelines will likewise enjoy civil immunity. See Morreim, "Cost Containment and the Standard of Medical Care," p. 1751.

37. I do not detail the plan here, for that is done elsewhere in this volume. Briefly, in 1989 the state of Oregon chose to expand its medicaid eligibility to cover all citizens below the poverty line instead of only the 58 percent then eligible. To accommodate so many more citizens within the same budget, the state instituted a plan for developing priorities by which to determine which health services would be covered. As the priority system developed, acute care of treatable life-threatening illnesses, such as bacterial pneumonia and peritonitis, topped the list of more than 700 different medical services and conditions. Toward the middle of the list were chronic diseases with treatments that could improve quality of life, such as multiple sclerosis and cerebral palsy. At the bottom were fatal illnesses for which there was little hope of improvement, such as advanced AIDS. See Diane S. Lund, "Oregon Panel Issues Updated Medicaid Priority Treatment List," *American Medical News*, March 11, 1991, pp. 1, 45, 46; and David C. Hadorn, "Setting Health Care Priorities in Oregon: Cost-Effectiveness Meets the Rule of Rescue," *Journal of the American Medical Association*, vol. 265 (May 1, 1991), pp. 2218–25. Each year the legislature must establish a level of funding and draw a line in the priority list to determine which sorts of care would be funded. In any given budget year, only the services ranked above, and none below, that year's priority level would be funded.

38. Ore. Rev. Stats. Ann. 414.745. While granting this immunity, Oregon also requires physicians to disclose openly to patients any instances in which the level of their care may be less than that which would usually be provided elsewhere. "Health care providers contracting to provide services . . . shall advise a patient of any service, treatment or test that is medically necessary but not covered under the contract if an ordinarily careful practitioner in the same or similar community would do so under the same or similar circumstances." Ore. Rev. Stats. Ann. 414.725(7).

39. Randall J. Bovbjerg, "Legislation on Medical Malpractice: Further Developments and a Preliminary Report Card," *University of California, Davis Law Review*, vol. 22 (1989), p. 1385.

40. Clark C. Havighurst, "Private Reform of Tort-Law Dogma: Market Opportunities and Legal Obstacles," *Law and Contemporary Problems*, vol. 49 (Spring 1986), pp. 143–72; Glen O. Robinson, "Rethinking the Allocation of Medical Malpractice Risks between Patients and Providers," *Law and Contemporary Problems*, vol. 49 (Spring 1986), pp. 173–200; Richard A. Epstein, "Medical Malpractice, Imperfect Information, and the Contractual Foundation for

Medical Services," *Law and Contemporary Problems*, vol. 49 (Spring 1986), pp. 201–12; Richard A. Epstein, "Medical Malpractice: The Case for Contract," *American Bar Foundation Research Journal*, vol. 1 (1976), pp. 87–149; and Clark C. Havighurst, "Altering the Applicable Standard of Care," *Law and Contemporary Problems*, vol. 49 (Spring 1986), pp. 265–76.

41. *Tunkl* v. *Regents of University of California*, 383 P.2d 411 (Cal. 1963); *Olson* v. *Molzen*, 558 S.W. 2d 429 (Tn. 1977); and *Wheeler* v. *St. Joseph Hospital*, 133 Cal. Rptr. 775 (Cal. App. 1977).

42. Indeed, in a system in which citizens can choose from many different packages with varying sorts of coverage, one can argue that each person is, in effect, choosing his own rationing system. Rather than impose a single rationing scheme on all citizens, a diversity of insurance options can enable each person to choose what works best for him. Some may wish to buy a comprehensive plan that covers everything from organ transplants to infertility treatments; others might want a leaner package, perhaps with high cost-sharing, so as to have more of their money available for other priorities. See Stuart M. Butler and Edmund F. Haislmaier, eds., *A National Health System for America* (Washington: Heritage Foundation, 1989). Arguably, such a choice-centered system would be most acceptable in the context of a national health plan that assures all citizens some basic minimum of care. In this way, no citizen would be medically neglected, nor, reciprocally, would anyone be permitted to be a "free rider" on the system by deliberately choosing an inadequate plan and then relying on others to provide him with appropriate care when he is in need. Citizens could choose options above the basic level, but no one would be required, or even permitted, to choose a clearly inadequate package. In such a system in which someone has made such a choice in the presence of ample information and options, he can rightly be expected to live with its consequences. He has chosen his own SRU and should accept the implications of his own choice. Some major changes would be expected to occur before such a system was implemented: a genuine variety of clearly described options, for example, instead of the endless petty variety that emerges from hundreds of concealed, idiosyncratic "cookbooks" that now guide various insurers' diverse definitions of medically necessary care. And full, complete information would have to be provided—not only about what each plan covers, but what it does not, and what sorts of incentives and controls it places on physicians and subscribers to contain costs. Even in a nonuniversal system, however, the law still expects parties in an insurance contract to conform to their agreement. When a patient has chosen to purchase care himself, he is expected to pay for it unless his physician has agreed to care for him gratuitously. In that sense, people can and do choose their own SRU. Admittedly, our current system does not always provide this level of choice and information. Still, when people have had the opportunity to enter knowledgeably

and voluntarily into a contract, the legal presumption is to enforce that contract.

43. *Sarchett v. Blue Shield of California*, 729 P. 2d 267 (Cal. 1987); and *Lockshin v. Blue Cross of Northeast Ohio*, 434 N.E. 2d 754 (Ohio App. 1980). For a contrasting minority view, see *Van Vactor v. Blue Cross Ass'n*, 365 N.E. 2d 638 (Ill. 1977).

44. *Dowd v. New York O. & W. Ry. Co.*, 63 N.E. 541 (N.Y. 1902); *Murphy v. Steeplechase Amusement Co.*, 166 N.E. 173 (N.Y. 1929); and *McEvoy v. City of New York*, 42 N.Y.S.2d 746 (N.Y. App. 1943), aff'd 55 N.E.2d 517 (N.Y. 1944).

45. *Schneider v. Revici*, 817 F.2d 987 (2nd Cir. 1987).

46. Ideally, one might prefer a health care system in which every person would (must) be insured, and every insurance package would include certain basic benefits. These requirements would ensure that society would not be burdened by "free riders" who chose to buy little or no coverage and then still expect full health care when in need. See Butler and Haislmaier, *A National System for America*.

47. Siliciano, "Wealth, Equity and the Unitary Medical Malpractice Standard," p. 439.

48. *Tunkl v. Regents of University of California*, 383 P.2d; *Olson v. Molzen*, 558 S.W. 2d; and *Wheeler v. St. Joseph Hospital*, 133 Cal. Rptr.

49. *Madden v. Kaiser Foundation Hospitals*, 552 P.2d 1178 (Cal. 1976).

50. Hirshfeld, "Tort Considerations for Third Party Payors."

51. *Wickline v. State of California*, 228 Cal. Rptr. 661 (Cal. App. 2 Dist. 1986). See also *Wilson v. Blue Cross of Southern Cal.*, 271 Cal. Rptr. 876 (Cal. App. 2 Dist. 1990).

52. Kenneth S. Abraham, "Judge-Made Law and Judge-Made Insurance: Honoring the Reasonable Expectations of the Insured," *Virginia Law Review*, vol. 67 (1981), p. 1168; and *McLaughlin v. Connecticut General Life Ins. Co.*, 565 F. Supp. 434 at 440 (Calif. 1983).

53. *Madden v. Kaiser Foundation Hospitals*, 552 P.2d at 1185; and *Wheeler v. St. Joseph Hospital*, 133 Cal. Rptr. at 783.

54. *Egan v. Mutual of Omaha Ins. Co.*, 598 P.2d 452 at 456 (Cal. 1979).

55. *Hughes v. Blue Cross of Northern Calif.*, 245 Cal. Rptr. 273 (Cal. App. 1988); and *Eichenseer v. Reserve Life Ins. Co.*, 881 F.2d 1355 (5th Cir. 1989).

56. Hirshfeld, "Tort Considerations for Third Party Payors," p. 83.

57. Ibid., p. 84.

58. *Maher v. Roe*, 432 U.S. at 469; *Harris v. McRae*, 448 U.S. at 301; and *Alexander v. Choate*, 105 S. Ct. at 722.

59. *Wilder v. Virginia Hosp. Ass'n*, 110 S.Ct. 2510 (Va. 1990).

60. *Greater Washington D.C. Area C. of SR. Cit. v. D.C. Government*, 406 F. Supp. 768 at 775 (1975).

61. Ibid. at 770.

62. Ibid. at 776.

63. *Boone* v. *Tate*, 286 A.2d 29 (Comm. Pa. 1972).

64. *Preston* v. *City of Philadelphia*, 362 A.2d 452 (Pa. Comm. 1976).

65. See pp. 166–69 in this paper, and *Alexander* v. *Choate*, 105 S. Ct. at 722.

66. Hadorn, "Setting Health Care Priorities in Oregon."

Justice and Health Care Rationing: Lessons from Oregon

Oregon's rationing plan has attracted two distinct audiences. In the United States, the plan is viewed by other states as a way to narrow the insurance gap without committing extensive new resources to health care. Outside the United States, the plan is considered a model for how universal access systems can determine which services are most important to provide as covered benefits. My initial remarks about equality are aimed at the plan's domestic uses; my comments on the rationing process are more general.

DISTINGUISHING MORAL FROM POLITICAL CRITICISMS OF THE OREGON PLAN

The Oregon Basic Health Services Act boldly couples the rationing of health care with a plan to improve access. Judged as a final product, the legislation is subject to important moral objections that I consider in the next three sections. According to Senator Kitzhaber, however, this legislation is only the beginning of an incremental strategy for more comprehensive reform of the system.[1] He intends to expand the plan to include the elderly on medicaid and medicare, and to extend the prioritization process to cover acute and long-term care over the lifespan. He also wants to offer the resulting insurance package to

This work was generously supported by grants from the National Endowment for the Humanities (RH-20917) and the National Library of Medicine (1RO1LM05005). Helpful information, materials, or comments were provided by Dan Brock, Arthur Caplan, Michael Garland, John Golenski, Bruce Jennings, and Paige Sipes-Metzler. Some material from this paper appeared in my article, "Is the Oregon Rationing Plan Fair?" *Journal of the American Medical Association*, vol. 265 (May 1, 1991), pp. 2232–35.

employers, which is directed toward a dominant or single-payer position for the public insurance scheme. The state could then bargain successfully to contain costs and could provide a way of capping health care costs in the state.

If the Oregon Plan is really part of an incremental strategy whose purpose is such comprehensive reform, then some moral criticisms of the plan, especially some of the points that are made about the inequities that the plan permits, apply only to its initial stages. Critics who have claimed the plan is "immoral" may actually share its proponents' goals and ultimate principles and disagree only with their political judgments about tactics and consequences. In a public debate, it is essential to distinguish moral disagreement about goals and principles from political disagreements about means. The following remarks target the existing legislation—not any long-term strategy based upon it.

RATIONING AND EQUALITY

Oregon explicitly rejects the rationing strategy that predominates in the United States, which excludes entire categories of the poor and near-poor from access to public insurance, and denies coverage to people rather than to low-priority services. In contrast, the Oregon Plan embodies the principle that maintains that there is a social obligation to guarantee universal access to a basic level of health care, which can be determined by a public process according to resource limitations.

This principle is not a complete account of justice for health care, but, as far as it goes, it has considerable plausibility, is widely accepted in the United States, and derives support from theoretical work on justice and health care. Disease and disability restrict an individual's range of opportunities, whereas health care, which maintains and restores normal functioning, protects individual opportunity.[2] Therefore, the health care system must be designed to protect equality of opportunity at each stage of life. This means there must be no financial or other discriminatory barriers to access to the level of health care that best promotes normal functioning and that best protects the range of opportunities open to individuals in that society. Because resources are limited, however, people are not entitled to every service that might potentially benefit them. Thus, society must develop fair procedures for meeting the most important needs, while respecting the moral principle of protecting equality of opportunity. The Oregon Plan violates this principle because it restricts rationing to the poorest groups in society. Justice is not opposed to rationing—indeed, it may require it—but justice imposes some egalitarian constraints on rationing, and these are not reflected in the Oregon Plan.

The Burden Borne by the Poor

Does the Oregon Plan exacerbate the condition of the poor? Consider the worst case, a zero-sum game with resources. For example, if some lower-priority services are removed and no higher-priority services, unavailable before the plan, are added, current medicaid recipients will lose some services and the health benefits they produce. They will no doubt then say, "We bear the burden of the plan. We are already the most indigent group, or close to it, so we should not have to give up important medical services so that the currently uninsured can get basic health care."

It is important to understand the moral force of this complaint. Notice that aggregate health status for all the poor, including current medicaid recipients and the uninsured, can be improved by the plan, although current medicaid recipients are made worse off. Losses to current recipients are more than counterbalanced by the gains of the uninsured, because the former lose less important services than the latter gain. As a result, the plan reduces overall inequality between the poor and the rest of society—albeit at the expense of current medicaid recipients. Because the barrier between current medicaid recipients and the currently uninsured is porous, not permanent, all the poor (working or not) have an interest in access to a basic health care package. Therefore, the complaint cannot be that the plan makes society less equal; instead, it is that even greater reductions in inequality are possible if other groups sacrifice instead of them. It is unfair for current medicaid recipients to bear a burden that others could bear much better—especially because inequality would then be even further reduced.

Consider next a scenario involving expanded resources. Suppose certain high-priority services were made more available, while low-ranked services were eliminated (which is the effect of the Oregon legislature's funding decisions in the spring of 1991). Current medicaid recipients may have a higher expected payoff from the plan—no one will be worse off, and aggregate inequality will be reduced even more. Nevertheless, current medicaid recipients can still say, "We achieved our gain in health status only by giving up beneficial services that other, better-off groups have not had to give up, and in that sense we bear the burden of the plan. All the poor could have been even better off if other groups had contributed more or other steps had been taken."

This complaint has force. By eliminating inefficiencies in our current system—such as by establishing a low-overhead public insurance scheme, as in Canada, or by developing treatment protocols that eliminate unnecessary services—we might be able to avoid making current medicaid recipients any worse off. Alternatively, by broadening rationing to cover most of society, as in Canada, Great Britain, and the Netherlands, we could avoid the criticism that only the poor are being made to bear the burden of improving access. Viewed as a final goal, the Oregon Plan is subject to moral criticisms that might not apply if the current legislation was followed by other reforms that extend the rationing to most of the population.

The Objectionable Structure of Inequality

Contrast the kind of inequality the Oregon Plan accepts with the inequality that arises in the heavily rationed British system. Although about 10 to 15 percent of the British public buys private insurance coverage to procure various rationed services, the overwhelming majority abides by the consequences of rationing. This produces a more acceptable *structure of inequality* than would result if the bottom 20 percent of the Oregon population ultimately has no access to some services that are available to the great majority.

To understand the reason that one structure of inequality seems worse than the other, consider how the poor would feel under both. Under the Oregon Plan, the poor can complain that society as a whole is content not only to leave them economically wanting but also to deny them medical services that would protect the range of opportunities open to them. There is a basis here for reasonable regrets or resentment by the poor, because society as a whole seems content to deny them the mainstream of opportunities. They may reasonably believe that such a division does not adequately respect their status as free and equal moral agents—if the majority really respected that status, it would not leave the poor with such disadvantages.[3] Alternatively, if health care protects opportunity in a way that is roughly equal for all, except that the most advantaged group has some extra advantages, then this may seem somewhat unfair, but no one group is then singled out for special disadvantages that are viewed as "acceptable" by the economically and medically advantaged majority. Consequently, no group would have a basis for the strong and reasonable regrets that the poor have under the Oregon Plan, despite the improvement over their current situation.

Thus, even if the poor are better off under the Oregon Plan than they now are, the plan still accepts an inequality that is not ideally just. It is more just—perhaps much more just—than what exists now, but still not what justice requires. Does this mean that we should not implement it? The answer seems to depend on political judgments about the feasibility of alternatives. If one thinks a uniform, universal plan, such as Canada's, is politically impossible in the United States, or if one thinks that introducing the Oregon Plan makes further reform in the direction of a uniform plan more likely (as in Kitzhaber's long-term strategy), then opting for the Oregon Plan, even if it is not ideally just, seems reasonable. But if one thinks that introducing the Oregon reform makes more radical reform of the system less likely, then one might well prefer not to make a modest improvement in the justice of the system in the interest of facilitating a more significant improvement later.

RATIONING AND FAIR PROCEDURES

The Oregon Plan also raises questions as to whether the procedures used to allocate resources are fair.

Advantage of Explicit Rationing

The Oregon Plan involves public, explicit, democratically accountable rationing; it disavows rationing hidden by the covert workings of a market or buried in the quiet, professional decisionmaking of providers—either at the bedside or in allocating resources within fixed hospital budgets. This insistence on publicity is controversial. In a celebrated work, Calabresi and Bobbitt argue that some "tragic choices" are best made away from public view in order to preserve important symbolic values, such as the sanctity of life.[4]

Despite the importance of protecting public symbols, however, justice would seem to require publicity. People who view themselves as free and equal moral agents must have available to them the rationale for the decisions that affect their lives in as fundamental a way as rationing would. Only with publicity can they resolve disputes about whether the decisions conform to the more basic principles of justice that are the accepted basis of their social cooperation.

Criticisms of the Community Meeting Process

Justice requires publicity and public accountability, not necessarily direct, participatory democracy. Especially when technical matters are involved, democratic theory requires only indirect representation. Direct participation, of course, might have some advantages in providing enhanced legitimation for the outcome—people are "directly consenting" to "self-imposed" constraints on their care—as well as education for those involved. Other states and some European countries like the idea of community participation, partly because they may have mistakenly believed the community was actually ranking services. Nevertheless, several objections can be made to the community meeting process.

First, the community meetings are too brief and their discussions are too superficial to develop a clear picture of community values. It takes hours of classroom discussion of subtly varied cases to clarify the values and principles that play a role in one medical choice or scenario—to say nothing about the many used by Oregon Health Decisions (OHD) in the community meetings. Second, the community meeting process is open to two charges of bias—the composition of the meetings was not representative of the population affected by the rationing plan, and the task assigned the meetings presupposes rationing only to the poor. The bias in the task magnifies the bias in composition, because we worry less about who is making a decision when it has an equal impact on everyone.

Third, the product of the meetings—an unranked list of thirteen "values"—cannot be used directly by the commissioners to rank procedures. Some of the values are merely categories of services that are underprovided in our system, such as prevention, mental health, and chemical dependency; others, such as equity, are properties of the system as a whole. Fourth, although the commissioners were influenced by values on the list when they ranked the seventeen general categories of treatments, the reason they weighted these values as they did is unclear. Thus, certain reproductive services and preventive services are given relatively high priority, which may be out of line either with their expected medical benefit or with some other "objective" measure of their payoff.

Finally, the fact that eleven Health Services commissioners—more than half of whom were health professionals—believed certain services were more important than others, in light of their interpretation of the evidence about community values, means that rankings were really the result of an indirect democratic process, not a participatory one as the press attention to the community meetings might have led us to believe. There is no reason to believe that a different set of commissioners, reacting to the same community meeting process, would have arrived at a similar ranking of services. The Oregon Health Services Commission (OHSC), despite the description it provided of the procedures that were followed in ranking categories, has offered no principled accounting of when or why it allowed an appeal to a community preference about services to outweigh evidence about the medical benefits of a service.

Unresolved Moral Issues in Ranking Procedures

Although the OHSC was charged to consider "community values" in ranking services, its initial methodology used a version of cost-effectiveness ranking involving Kaplan's quality-of-well-being scale. There is no plausible way to integrate the result of community meetings with such a methodology. When the "infamous" computer-generated cost-effectiveness rankings of June 1990 appeared, they were quickly subjected to ridicule for the counterintuitive or anomalous priorities they contained. For example, appendectomy ranked lower than tooth capping because the greater medical benefit of appendectomy was outweighed by the lower cost of tooth capping.[5] This violated what Hadorn calls "The Rule of Rescue," which requires us to give priority to lifesaving services; a more plausible and general rule of rescue might require giving priority to treating more serious (disabling) conditions over less serious ones, whether or not they were life threatening.

Because of the anomalies cost-effectiveness ranking produced, the OHSC revised the prioritization procedure. Commissioners ranked seventeen general categories of condition-treatment pairs—thus, life-saving services that fully restore normal functioning were given priority over nonlifesaving services or services that did not fully restore normal functioning. Cost was considered only within categories, and any remaining "anomalies" were subject to "hand adjustment." Reproductive services (excluding infertility), preventive medical services, and dental services were given priority over some medical or surgical treatments for various serious, but not fatal, conditions; infertility treatments were given low priority.

On what basis were these hand adjustments made? Was the placement of these categories influenced by the commissioners' perceptions of community values, or by their responses to effective "logrolling" by special interest groups? What is clear, in any case, is that these rankings violate the more general, modified Rule of Rescue.

There are deeper moral grounds for criticizing these rankings. The OHSC ranking of categories does not respect the relative importance of services that maintain or restore normal functioning. The rankings are, therefore, not proportional to their effect on the range of opportunities open to individuals. For example, tooth cleaning and tubal ligation are ranked higher than hip replacement, even though the disability produced by hip degeneration far more seriously impairs the functioning and, thus, opportunities open to individuals than either tooth caries or the need to use other forms of birth control does. Similarly, vasectomy is ranked higher than infertility treatment, although the impairment of opportunity produced by infertility is far greater than the inconvenience that results from using alternative forms of male contraception. The Oregon rankings' failure to reflect the impact on opportunity is shared by other prominent methodologies. For example, as has been seen, cost-effectiveness rankings will override effects on opportunity. Similarly, ranking services by expected medical benefit—whether it is done by condition-treatment pairs, as in Oregon, or by a more detailed analysis that considers the specific condition of each patient—has the problematic consequence that higher priority will be given to patients who have a high probability of correcting a less serious impairment than to those who have a lower probability of correcting a more serious condition. Of course, sometimes such an outcome is preferable. Resources should not be directed toward cases in which only marginal improvement is possible. But in other instances, ignoring the patient who is more seriously impaired in favor of one with a less serious disease or disability seems unacceptable, despite what the methodology tells us about expected benefits. How to draw a reasonable line here is the main unresolved issue facing those who must make rationing decisions. It is clearly a problem left unsolved by the Oregon procedure.

In contexts where there is no clear consensus or conclusive moral arguments that favor a particular principle for determining a fair outcome, a fair procedure may have to be relied upon. That may be the best that can be done in the case of ranking the importance of medical procedures. The outcome of such a process is not sacred, however, and it must be subject to criticism based on moral and methodological arguments aimed at negotiating improvements in solving the ranking problem. The OHSC rankings are prime targets for such criticism.

Political Pressures and the Legislature

Political judgments obviously diverge on how much the legislature can be trusted. The crucial issue from the point of view of process, however, is this: because the Oregon Plan explicitly involves rationing primarily for the poor and near poor, funding decisions face constant political pressure from more powerful groups that want to put public resources to other uses. In contrast, if the legislature were deciding how to fund a rationing plan that applied to themselves and to all or most of their constituents, then one might expect a careful and honest weighing of the importance of health care against other goods. The legislature would then have stronger reasons not to concede to political pressures to divert resources, and other groups would be less likely to apply such pressure. If the plan is expanded to include other groups, as some proponents intend, then the poor may find important allies. In systems like the Canadian or Dutch, where rationing would apply either to everyone or to a significant majority, the concern about the voting power of the poor is less serious (indeed, the existence of those systems suggests that the poor have greater voting power in those societies).

The chief worries about fairness in the Oregon rationing process derive from its being aimed at the poor rather than at the entire population. Concerns about fairness in the process thus converge with concerns about the kinds of inequality the system tolerates. This does not mean that the Oregon experiment should not be tried, for it may produce less overall inequality in health status than now exists. It should be recognized from the start, however, that a system that rations only to the poor is less equitable than alternative systems that ration for most people. To the extent that the inequality ultimately troubles many participants in the system, including physicians who will be able to do only certain things for some children and more for others, the strains of commitment to abiding by the rationing will be greater, and rationing may get a worse name than it deserves.

CONCLUSION

The Oregon Plan retains its structure of inequality because states must respond to the problems imposed by a highly inequitable and highly inefficient national health care system. The plan contains a bizarre irony. The state medicaid budget is in crisis because of rapidly increasing costs—most of which are the results of the long-term-care burden imposed by the elderly—yet, the rationing plan focuses on poor children. Oregon did not design a medicaid system that forces the most vulnerable children and the most vulnerable elderly to compete for scarce public resources. As long as states must respond to problems created by the national system, however, their solutions will inherit its major flaws. Uncoordinated responses by states cannot solve the problems caused by the continuing rapid dissemination of technology, inefficiencies in administering a mixed system, and a growing demand for services in our aging and AIDS-ridden society.

Reasonable people may differ in their political judgments about whether the Oregon Plan is a useful steppingstone to a more equitable rationing scheme or whether it delays more radical and more equitable reforms of the health care system, such as a Canadian-style system. Oregon's commitment to provide universal access to basic care and to make rationing a subject of open, political debate should be welcomed. But the country should not settle for a plan that accepts the kinds of unjustifiable inequality the Oregon Plan permits. More work must be done to solve the moral and methodological problems involved in ranking the importance of medical services, because Oregon's procedure is far from ideal.

NOTES

1. John Kitzhaber, president of the Oregon Senate, personal communication, January and February 1991.

2. Norman Daniels, *Just Health Care* (Cambridge University Press, 1985), chap. 3; and Norman Daniels, *Am I My Parents' Keeper? An Essay on Justice between the Young and the Old* (Oxford University Press, 1988), chap. 4.

3. Joshua Cohen, "Democratic Equality," *Ethics*, vol. 99 (1989), pp. 727–51; and Thomas M. Scanlon, "Contractualism and Utilitarianism" in Amartya Sen and Bernard Williams, eds., *Utilitarianism and Beyond* (Cambridge University Press, 1982), pp. 103–28.

4. Guido Calabresi and Philip Bobbitt, *Tragic Choices* (Norton, 1978).

5. David Hadorn, "Setting Health Care Priorities in Oregon: Cost-Effectiveness Meets the Rule of Rescue," *Journal of the American Medical Association*, vol. 265 (May 1, 1991), pp. 2218–25.

H. TRISTRAM ENGELHARDT, JR.

Why a Two-Tier System of Health Care Delivery Is Morally Unavoidable

The public policy challenge is to create health care policy, given three significant clusters of encumbrances. First, there is the desire on the part of most people to postpone death indefinitely; to lower the risk of suffering, disease, and disability; to ameliorate their suffering due to disease and disability; and not to spend so much on satisfying the first three desires as not to have enough resources left over to enjoy their lives. Second, there are only limited resources available to achieve the many projects that appeal to humans. Last and most important, there is no generally justifiable secular moral vision concerning justice, fairness, or the final significance and meaning of human life that will enable secular societies to discover how they should rank the first four desires.

The proposed Oregon Plan provides a heuristic for resolving the public policy challenge. The creation of a basic adequate package through communal funds can be regarded as a prudent act of self-insurance, as a limited act of solidarity with others, or as a limited act of altruism. These and probably other reasons and goals will motivate citizens to create a basic package whose secular authority will be derived from a communal decision. The existence of a private luxury tier, supported through private insurance and direct out-of-pocket payments, represents a recognition of the limits of communal authority to define the proper ways in which justice and fairness ought to be achieved; the right of individuals to deploy their private resources and energies as they wish, once they have discharged their limited civic duties; and the diversity of human values with regard to health, disease, health care, and the avoidance of risks.

THE FALLACIES OF ARGUMENTS
FOR EQUALITY

By accepting two-tier health care with a robust private tier,* the Oregon Plan builds implicitly on the 1983 report of the President's Commission for the Study of Ethical Problems in Medicine and Biomedical and Behavioral Research. That report dismissed the option of equity as equality in health care, in favor of "equity as an adequate level of health care."[1] By equity as equality, the report appears to mean a national health service or insurance scheme in which every citizen has the same level of health protection; by equity as the provision of an adequate level of care, the report appears to include plans that guarantee everyone a basic level of health care but allow inequalities in the level of health coverage.

Many social theorists, including Norman Daniels and Representative Sanders, do not accept the President's Commission's rejection of equity as equality and the consequent endorsement of equity as an adequate or basic level of health care. Moreover, they do not recognize that the pursuit of equality is constrained by substantial limits on public moral authority. In their view, an ultimate objective of public policy ought to be "equality." They reject "market policies" or other deviations from this standard unless the market is obviously more efficient than alternative means of distribution with respect to achieving their "canonical" ideals of equality. The main difficulty in this approach is that there are as many theories of justice, fairness, rights to health care, proper equality in health care, and the significance of individual preferences and of liberty as there are major religions. Moreover, there is no single, canonical, content-full, secular account of fairness, justice, and rights in health care that does not beg cardinal moral questions.†

The problem for a canonical, content-full, secular morality can be stated fairly succinctly, though the issues are fundamental and their consequences dramatic. Imagine that one were to agree that the four major goals to be achieved through social organization are liberty,

---

*I use the *two-tier health care system* to designate a system that has both a governmentally supported tier of health care and a privately financed tier. Each of these tiers may itself be composed of diverse segments or tiers.

†A theory is "content-full" if it incorporates or justifies a ranking of goods such as liberty and equality.

equality, prosperity, and security. Depending on how one decides to rank these four desiderata, one will be living either in North Korea or in Texas. The problem is how to rank fundamental moral goals. One cannot use Rawls's theory of justice or other hypothetical social contract theories to resolve this problem without already having decided, implicitly or explicitly, the crucial issue of ranking.[2] An appeal to hypothetical decisionmakers or contractors can establish a theory of justice only if one already possesses some particular moral sense or some "thin" theory of the good. The appeal to disinterested moral observation to establish a theory of justice for social policy is useless for moral issues, because it provides no grounds for choosing among alternative moral worlds. An observer who can choose, however, has already been rendered parochial by being fitted out with someone's particular moral sense or someone's particular thin theory of the good. The same problem arises in appeals to consequences or utilitarian considerations.[3] One must first know how to rank liberty-consequences, equality-consequences, security-consequences, and prosperity-consequences before one can calculate and compare the consequences associated with different approaches to distributing health care resources. For that matter, appeals to preferences will not work, either, because one must first know how to rank present preferences versus future preferences or rationally considered preferences versus impassioned preferences. The point is that one cannot discover which among the various rival accounts of justice and fairness one ought rationally to endorse, without already knowing the answer to the question—that is, without begging the central question about the proper content of morality, justice, or fairness.[4] One must first specify to whose justice or to which sense of moral rationality one is appealing to resolve a moral controversy.[5] But such a specification renders the outcome parochial and limited in moral governance.

Despite the limitations of secular moral reason, people often seem disposed to make substantial moral claims. For example, once ill, many people feel that their unfortunate circumstance is more than simply unfortunate and that the fates or the gods have dealt unfairly with them. Many such persons hold it to be not simply fortunate for others, but also unfair that those others have remained healthy, or that others have set aside or acquired funds that allow them to purchase health care that may extend life or render life more comfortable, while they lack these resources. At this point, an important fallacy has been committed: the fallacy of confounding the unfortunate with the unfair.[6] Because in secular terms we are not responsible for, nor do we merit, the blessings and banes of fate, we cannot recognize them as our due. The results of fate are neither merited nor unmerited. They are there in the sense that, aside from theological understandings or revelations, they are neither fair nor unfair. But once one comes to possess certain benefits owing to fate, that they are unmerited does not make those benefits any less one's own. Nor does it undercut one's claim to enjoy them.

Consider what it would be like if you helped a stranger solve a mathematical problem. Once you provide the solution in the absence of prior claims, the benefits belong to the stranger. It is neither fair nor unfair that the stranger has them, enjoys them, or gives them or sells them to others. It is, however, fortunate for the stranger. Conversely, if the stranger suffers an illness, that is merely unfortunate, not unfair. Against this background, those who attempt to expand the scope of basic coverage can be regarded as appealing to an egalitarianism of altruism (that is, attempting to advantage the disadvantaged by providing them more), while those who wish to forbid those who can from buying more treatment can be regarded as appealing to an egalitarianism of jealousy (that is, not aiming at raising the status of the disadvantaged but at lowering the status of the advantaged).

THE MORAL PRETENSIONS OF ETHICISTS AND ECONOMISTS

Despite the limits of secular moral reasoning, many economists, ethicists, and bioethicists act as though there were no great difficulties with their positions. They come, as it were, as priests and priestesses of different sets of canonical moral intuitions and assumptions. They forward their particular intuitions and assumptions as though they ought to be endorsed by all rational men and women. They rarely declare, "I am about to give you an account of certain intuitions of fairness and justice which you are likely to share if you identify with a particular ideological or philosophical tradition." Or perhaps, "I am about to give you an account of certain intuitions of fairness and justice which you are likely to endorse as a modern Western yuppie who votes left of center." Or better yet, "I hope to convert you to the only moral vision that I believe should be endorsed by humans." Instead, they advance their intuitions as though they were to be endorsed by people who do not subscribe to any particular moral tradition. To forestall misunderstandings, one must realize that there is no single canonical American tradition or understanding of the American way. One need only compare the competing visions of the American tradition as endorsed by Ronald Reagan, Michael Dukakis, and the Libertarian candidate Ron Paul.

Often, discussions regarding the proper allocation of health care resources turn on amazing assumptions about particular canonical intuitions. Proponents of particular views of justice in general, and of justice in health care allocation in particular, advance conflicting possible moral worlds and then ask their interlocutors to choose in an attempt to disclose background canonical moral intuitions. For example, consider the choice between a world of health care resource allocation in which there are one hundred people, eighty of whom have ten health care utiles (units of utility) each and twenty of whom have only four health care utiles each, and a world with a hundred people, all of whom have six health care utiles each (it is presumed in all other matters these worlds are equal). In the second world, there is less average and total utility than in the first (for example, 600 total utiles versus 880), but there is equality. There is no longer a less advantaged group that has less than the rest. Often, at this juncture, people are asked about their intuitions, about how they feel or intuit about equality, fairness, and maximization of utility, in an attempt to establish a particular canonical moral viewpoint. How could one ever discover which intuitions are the rationally canonical? Does one simply appeal to what is currently in moral fashion?

If the answer is affirmative, then one should recognize that the economists, ethicists, or bioethicists who support such appeals to current fashion are not playing the paradigmatic role of the ethicist within the aspirations of modern moral philosophy—namely, to provide an account of what rational individuals as such ought morally to endorse. Each is trying to aver, more convincingly than the other, a particular set of intuitions, or the moral fashion of a particular moral community, so as then to take the leap of faith and conclude which intuitions and mores must bind and should bind rational persons as such. Or, to put the matter somewhat more unkindly, they may be engaged in ideological proselytizing or in political propaganda hidden under the cloak of general secular reason.

Here it is important to distinguish between the strong role and the weak role of economists, ethicists, and bioethicists, where strength and weakness are defined in terms of the capacity to deliver concrete moral canons for human behavior that should govern persons as such, apart from particular allegiances to particular cultural traditions. The more that the strong role can be realized, the more it should be possible to provide a general justification for an all-encompassing health care system by securing a foundational account of justice or fairness. The more one is skeptical of the feasibility of such a project, the more the "market rationing" of health care turns out to be appropriate by default. When one cannot justify the authority to intervene coercively, persons are at liberty—not because one values liberty, but because would-be coercers cannot give a moral justification for their interventions.

THE MORAL CENTRALITY OF THE MARKET

It is important to distinguish market rationing from nonmarket rationing. Market rationing is distribution of energies and goods through the free choice of individuals and groups as a result of their own decisions. Nonmarket rationing is distribution through the imposition of a particular pattern or mode for the allocation of goods and services. The first does not require a person to secure any claims regarding the proper, fair, just, or morally appropriate way in which goods and resources ought to be distributed, nor does it involve the claim that a third party, such as a government, has the moral authority to impose a particular pattern, however discovered or created. It is for this reason that most people do not ordinarily consider market distribution to be rationing.

Still, both market and nonmarket modes of distribution can be understood as occurring according to a principle. In the market, distribution occurs according to the principle of mutual agreement. In nonmarket rationing, distribution is made according to an imposed pattern or procedure other than the agreement of the parties to the exchange. In each case, there is a reason for the way things are distributed. But the *ratio* or reason is quite different in the two instances. In the market, one need not claim that one knows how things ought to be distributed. One need not claim that markets distribute things best or most efficiently. One need only claim that people are at liberty to choose how to exchange their own goods and services. It is because of this straightforward, nonmetaphysical justification that market transactions are generally so unproblematic. Market rationing, in short, makes few demands on reason to discover content-full canonical moral guidelines. It does not require reason to discover the proper pattern of distribution. The most fundamental justification for the market rationing of health care services is that no one has the secular moral authority to forbid it. That is, because of their moral limitations, secular states do not have the moral authority to forbid individuals to purchase health care either directly or through private insurance.

All-encompassing nonmarket rationing (one that does not allow a private tier) presupposes that individuals are so owned by, or subject to the authority of, others—such as their society or government— that a particular pattern for the distribution of their own goods and services may be imposed despite their wishes to the contrary. To justify all-encompassing nonmarket rationing morally, one would wish to show that one knows what the proper distribution of resources ought to be, that one has the authority to impose it on the unconsenting over their protests, and that the imposition will effect more benefit than harm. As has been argued above, there is no content-full canonical vision of distributive justice or equality that may be imposed in an all-encompassing fashion. The unavoidable conclusion, therefore, is that market rationing is most closely compatible with a pluralistic secular democracy. The centrality of individuals as the source of secular authority is therefore not a function of some special value given to individuals or to individual freedom. It is simply that real individuals are all we have as a starting point for fashioning secular projects. The basis for the moral centrality of a market in health care is that the market gains its authority from the consent of those who engage in trading goods for health care services.

THE MORAL SIGNIFICANCE OF OREGON

The importance of the Oregon proposal is that it recognizes two cardinal constraints. First, it forthrightly acknowledges the moral unavoidability of a private tier of health care in which health care can be purchased directly or by private insurance. In so doing, the Oregon proposal considers a fundamental moral truth—namely, the moral limits of a secular democracy. Absent an authoritative divine decree and absent what contemporary philosophy has failed to provide (that is, a canonical content-full account of justice), men and women are left to the device of creating limited common projects with limited moral authority, and are constrained to eschew the notion that citizens, their property, and their services are wholly owned by the society or state. One is left with the rather straightforward claim that after people have paid their taxes, they may take their remaining resources and purchase whatever they wish, whether that is philosophy books or additional health care.

Second, the Oregon approach acknowledges that a broad constituency exists for creating from common funds a basic, adequate package of health care for all citizens. One need not be able to disclose God's will, or the content-full constraints of a canonical view of justice, to fashion a basic health care package democratically. Moreover, insofar as God is silent (that is, is not heard unambiguously by all), and insofar as many equally plausible theories of justice and of rights to health care remain, citizens will need to decide democratically what they will do with their common resources, while not acting as though all resources were commonly owned. Oregon's approach to health care involves the straightforward recognition that citizens must consider how much of their common resources they wish to set aside for health care, and which health care goods and services they wish to purchase.

On this second point, Oregon provides an excellent example of a society confronting the cultural challenge of coming to terms with human finitude in the face of the hubris often engendered by health care technology. Because all of life is a gamble, and because medicine is part of life, there will be more or less certain wagers of resources on technological innovations to gain a particular health benefit. There will never be enough money to use all the available technological expedients to avoid all the risks of death and disability, given competing interests. As a result, individuals and societies will use some, not all, of what modern medicine offers. Having set aside funds for some, but not all, medical interventions, one will need to live with two outcomes. First, people will die because resources were not set aside to avoid some risks of death and disability. Second, those who have sufficient funds may still be able to purchase additional medical interventions and survive while others die. The second outcome in health care is something like outcomes in other areas of life, such as with the fortunate persons who can buy those more crash-resistant cars that far exceed the basic requirements for crash safety and therefore survive, while another 50,000 or so die in the United States every year in automobile crashes because they do not have such protection.

Oregon helps its citizens confront the challenge of containing health care costs in the face of infinite expectations, through what is tantamount to a limited social insurance system. The democratic discussion that has framed the Oregon approach has encouraged an explicit articulation of a limited communal solidarity. The insurance model offers a means for people to think through, in advance of their actual need for health care, what type and scope of health care they want. Among other things, the insurance model or metaphor reminds people (1) that in creating a public health care system they are fashioning a limited social commitment of limited moral authority and scope, and (2) that the limits of that social commitment may not be expanded for particular persons in need by particular physicians or institutions without violating the conditions of the prior social agreement (of course, this prior condition would not preclude using funds from private sources).[7]

The Oregon Plan provides in its most general outline a heuristic procedure for health care policy debates. It is an attempt to address real-life moral concerns regarding health care in the face of finite moral and philosophical resources. It is the general elements of the Oregon Plan that must be underscored rather than particular elements of the current proposal. Oregon represents the first substantial attempt to democratize discussions regarding health care allocations. Despite the shortcomings that may beset the plan, Oregon has done better than any other state, or the federal government, in involving citizens as colleagues in the communal project of deciding how much to give to health care and what health care to purchase. Perhaps these debates are so complex that the federal government is systematically incapable of undertaking them with the seriousness and attention to communal concerns that have marked the Oregon debate.

In any event, one should take advantage of the fact that the United States were fashioned as a federation of sovereign states, providing the opportunity for each state to attempt to meet the challenge of framing a basic health care package. Because we have just begun to confront the cultural and financial costs of high-technology medicine, we would be well advised not to rush to embrace a national health care plan but to explore as many possible approaches as our patience and good sense allow us. If anything, the temptation will be to establish a final, complete, and encompassing solution for all the states, barely three decades into our experience with high-technology medicine. It is necessary to explore the different ways in which men and women can educate themselves about the problem of deploying finite resources in the face of both infinite expectations and limited moral authority. In all of this, the most important point to emphasize is Oregon's acknowledgement of the obvious fact that only citizens can determine how much of their communal resources should be deployed for health care, and how it should be used.[8]

The Oregon Plan recognizes what Canada fails to acknowledge—namely, the robust limits of secular limited democracies. The existence of a substantial private-tier health care represents a recognition of the limited authority of secular societies. After it has been decided how to dispense public funds for communal resources in creating a limited social insurance against health losses, people should be free to purchase additional health care according to their inclinations and resources. A private health care tier that is supported by private insurance, as well as by out-of-pocket expenditures, is important—not because of what it accomplishes, but because it acknowledges the limits of community authority and the diversity of individual moral sentiments and wishes.

NOTES

1. President's Commission for the Study of Ethical Problems in Medicine and Biomedical and Behavioral Research, *Securing Access to Health Care* (Government Printing Office, 1983), vol. 1, p. 20. The commission argued that one could not forbid a second tier of health care because "trying to prevent such inequalities would require interfering with people's liberty to use their income to purchase an important good like health care while leaving them free to use it for frivolous or inessential ends. Prohibiting people with higher incomes or stronger preferences for health care from purchasing more care than everyone else gets would not be feasible, and would probably result in a black market for health care" (pp. 18–19).

2. See John Rawls, *A Theory of Justice* (Harvard University Press, 1971); and Norman Daniels, *Just Health Care* (Cambridge University Press, 1985).

3. For a well-developed utilitarian argument for equality in health care distributions, see Peter Singer, "Freedoms and Utilities in the Distribution of Health Care," in Robert M. Veatch and Roy Branson, eds., *Ethics and Health Policy* (Ballinger, 1976), pp. 175–93. Similar considerations have been advanced in defense of the Canadian health care system. See, for instance, Robert G. Evans, "Health Care in Canada: Patterns of Funding and Regulation," *Journal of Health Politics, Policy and Law*, vol. 8 (Spring 1983), pp. 1–43.

4. It does not appear possible to provide a general rational foundation for a content-full moral philosophy by which to secure a content-full secular bioethics. See H. T. Engelhardt, Jr., *The Foundations of Bioethics* (Oxford University Press, 1986).

5. The confrontation with many alternative accounts of justice and moral rationality without a clear account of how one should choose among them defines the postmodern condition. Many authors have addressed this fragmentation of moral vision. See, for example, three books by Alasdair MacIntyre, published by Notre Dame University Press: *After Virtue* (1981), *Whose Justice? Which Rationality?* (1988), and *Three Rival Versions of Moral Enquiry* (1990); Richard Rorty, *Contingency, Irony, and Solidarity* (Cambridge University Press, 1989); and Kenneth Baynes, James Bohman, and Thomas McCarthy, eds., *After Philosophy* (MIT Press, 1987). See also H. T. Engelhardt, Jr., and A. L. Caplan, *Scientific Controversies* (Cambridge University Press, 1987).

6. See, for example, H. Tristram Engelhardt, Jr., *Bioethics and Secular Humanism: The Search for a Common Morality* (Philadelphia and London: Trinity Press International/SCM Press, 1991). See also H. Tristram Engelhardt, Jr., and Michael A. Rie, "Intensive Care Units, Scarce Resources, and Conflicting Principles of Justice," *Journal of the American Medical Association*, vol. 255 (March 7, 1986), pp. 1159–64.

7. Only if these two limitations are accepted can health care costs be contained within the bounds of a limited democracy. When confronted with the fact that they will die because they cannot afford a high-technology intervention that offers some possible benefit, patients too often react by either demanding that they be provided the treatment, even though the agreed-upon insurance does not provide it, or demanding that because they cannot afford the treatment, those who have the funds to purchase the treatment in question not be allowed to purchase the treatment, either.

8. Some people have considered the Oregon approach to be dangerous, in that it encourages citizens to consider how much they wish to tax themselves to provide a basic package of health care as well as to consider which health care services they would want to purchase. Such criticisms make sense if one presumes there are people in a secular society who are moral experts and can declare what God or reason requires to be expended for health care. Absent such assumptions, one may believe it is best to have members of Congress,

rather than citizens in the several sovereign states or members of state legislatures, face these important decisions. There are no good data to show, however, that members of Congress are less venal or wiser in this matter than
either members of state legislatures or the citizens of Oregon. Considering
the timidity of members of Congress in facing the obvious—namely, that
there must be a limit on how much money will be communally set aside to
save the lives of Americans—one might in general think much more highly of
the legislators and citizens of Oregon. In any event, in a matter as complex as
this, it would seem ideal to have fifty concurrent discussions and experiments
regarding the project of creating a basic adequate level of health care for all.

The Inevitability of Health Care Rationing: A Case Study of Rationing in the British National Health Service

The manifest intent of the Oregon health care reform initiative is to provide universal access to health care. To this end, the initiative mandates that employers provide their employees with basic health insurance coverage; it sets up a state insurance pool to cover those who are otherwise uninsurable; and unlike the medicaid program it will replace, it provides basic health insurance coverage for *everyone* below the poverty level.[1] Because retired people in Oregon receive health insurance through medicare, the effect of the initiative is to provide every citizen of the state with basic health insurance. But as the papers in this book attest, though this achievement has not gone unnoticed, it has not been the focus of public and scholarly commentary. What has riveted attention is that the basic health insurance coverage mandated by the Oregon reform uses a formal process that explicitly rations access to health care.

This paper explores the relationship between rationing and the nonmarket provision of health care by focusing on a single well-researched case in which universal access created problems of rationing—the British National Health Service. The BNHS is often characterized as "the most egalitarian [health care delivery system] in any industrialized country" and is undoubtedly the paradigmatic Western example of a conscious attempt to remove the market from the provision of health care.[2] In recent years, however, the BNHS has been cited as a conspicuous example of the discrepancy between initial egalitarian hopes for nonmarket health care provision and the eventual inegalitarian reality of such systems. The argument advanced here is that the experience of the BNHS shows that nonmarket health care delivery will not be egalitarian unless it replicates three crucial market functions: value prioritization, resource generation, and demand limitation. Thus, one moral drawn from this case study is that even nonmarket health delivery systems must "ration." A second moral is that when nonmarket health care delivery systems fail to openly and explicitly recognize the inevitability of rationing, they are forced to introduce covert, invisible rationing mechanisms. These mechanisms, however, violate formal constraints of justice and thus (the third moral) tend to institutionalize inequities. The final moral follows from the first three: as a matter of public policy, health care delivery systems should eschew invisible rationing mechanisms in favor of open, visible, explicit, direct rationing—as proposed in the Oregon initiative.

THE SEMANTICS OF "RATIONING"

Rationing is an emotionally charged term; many scholars, especially those favorably disposed to market economics, define it in such a way that market allocations never ration.[3] There is an etymological rationale for this narrow usage. *Ration* goes back to the Latin, *ratio*, which means reasoning or calculating. Moreover, the literal meaning of the English noun *ration* is *a share*—hence, the implication that a *ration* is a calculated share. The verb form, *to ration*, however, is often more broadly defined as *any* mechanism for allocating resources (including the market) in contexts in which demand (or need) is not completely satisfied—that is, any mechanism of allocation under conditions of scarcity.[4] In this paper *rationing* is used in the latter broad sense—to facilitate comparisons between market and nonmarket *rationing* mechanisms and to minimize the use of such jargon as *demand curtailment*.[5]

UNIVERSAL ACCESS AND RATIONING: THE CASE OF THE BNHS

Today, the initials BNHS are often taken to mean "British National Health Shortages." Nothing could have been further from the minds of the founders of the British National Health Service. On July 5, 1948, or the "appointed day," as it came to be called, the British Labour government took direct control of British health insurance funds, clinics, and hospitals in an attempt, to quote the words of Minister of Health Aneurin Bevin, to "universalize the best." The founders believed their endeavor could be financed with only a modest infusion of new funds, because the market system being replaced was inherently irrational and inefficient. Its irrationality was manifest in such redundancies as multiple private insurance companies; its inefficiencies were largely a function of a bias toward expensive emergency and acute care, rather than relatively inexpensive preventive and primary care. Hence, once the government rationalized the system (to quote a now famous line from the Beveridge Report of 1942),[6] "[The cost of] further development of the service would be offset by the fall in demand which would take place once the original backlog of need had been wiped out and the population became healthier as a result of better medical care, so that costs would not rise in subsequent years."[7]

Within four months of the "appointed day," however, the government discovered that it was in error. As Bevin wrote the cabinet, "The rush for spectacles, as for dental treatment, has exceeded all expectations. . . . Part of what has happened has been a natural first flush of the new scheme, with the feeling that everything is free now and it does not matter what is charged up to the Exchequer."[8]

By the spring of 1951, despite a 75 percent increase in funding, the situation had still not improved, and the government decided to balance its budget by imposing a fee for dentistry, drugs, and eyeglasses. The surcharge blatantly violated the principle of free health service, and Bevin resigned in protest.[9] In all, the BNHS experiment with unlimited, unrationed access to health care lasted a little less than three years.

Underlying the government's miscalculations was a failure to appreciate that markets not only equilibrate demand but (by sleight of Adam Smith's invisible hand) also generate a supply sufficient to meet it. In so doing (as Tristram Engelhardt argues elsewhere in this volume), individual decisions expressed through the market automatically order and prioritize values. The Labour government understood neither blade of Alfred Marshall's scissors (that is, the supply and demand curves) when it founded the BNHS. Not unnaturally, therefore, it failed to appreciate that in abolishing market provision of health care, it also eliminated a functioning mechanism for prioritizing values, for limiting demand, and for generating resources to increase supply. Failing to understand what it had eliminated, the government made no provision for any substitute in its plans for the BNHS—nor has a satisfactory substitute ever evolved, which is to say that, for its entire history, the BNHS has been in a state of financial crisis.

Another factor underlying the BNHS perpetual financial crisis was a misconception of the economic impact of increasing access to life-saving interventions. Death always economizes on direct health care delivery costs, since it ends a person's career as a consumer of health care. Increased access to lifesaving interventions, therefore, usually *increases* the direct cost of health care delivery—an effect exacerbated by the halfway nature of many lifesaving technologies (such as dialysis machines) that save life without completely restoring health. Thus, *if* the Beveridge Report was correct in presuming that financial barriers effectively denied many people access to modern scientific medicine and new lifesaving technologies, it should properly have concluded that removing these barriers would *increase* the direct cost of health care. Instead, it concluded precisely the opposite (as, indeed, do many contemporary commentators—despite the evidence of the historical record).

The mediated nature of health care consumption was another complicating factor. When professionals are permitted to act without constraint, they attempt to ensure that every patient, even those with relatively minor deviations from idealized norms, is restored to ideal health—perfect vision, form-fitting dentures, and so forth. The 1950 surcharges reinserted patients' financial concerns into the mediated decisionmaking process, which moderated professionals' inclinations to achieve ideal health for their patients. Reinstituting price, however, also replicated the very feature of the market provision of health care that was considered most unjust. The resulting political fiasco taught the BNHS to forgo the use of price as a mechanism for controlling mediated demand—ultimately leading it to an alternative expedient, training physicians to demand "less than the best" for their patients.

RATIONALIZATION AND RATIONING IN THE BNHS

At the same time that it reintroduced fees to fund "excessive" demand for dentures, drugs, and eyeglasses, the British government capped the total 1949–50 net budget for the BNHS.[10] Capping was as effective a cost constraint as surcharges; it soon became apparent that it had the additional advantage of being uncontentious—no one appeared to object to, or even take particular notice of, the budget caps. From that point onward, BNHS budgets were capped at the cabinet level. Regions and districts were directed to operate within fixed budgets and to accommodate increased demand for services by "rationalizing," to use the rhetoric of the day. Harry Eckstein, author of one of the first books on the BNHS, characterizes the ethos of rationalizing as follows. "'Rationalizing' in this context . . . implies, first, the economical organization of the services: the elimination of waste and duplication, the performance of medical functions where they are most suitably performed, and stretching existing personnel and facilities as far as possible by proper coordination and proper distribution of workloads."[11]

Rationalizing favored primary care as the least expensive form of health care delivery. Correlatively, there developed within the BNHS a systemic bias against the more expensive nonprimary care services: acute care (such as surgery), domiciliary chronic care (such as nursing homes and psychiatric hospitals), emergency care (such as shock-trauma centers), and above all else, tertiary care (such as intensive care units). Forty years of rationalizing left two prominent marks on the nonprimary care services: undercapitalization and waiting lists. Both were manifest to the naked eye; for until the Thatcher reforms of the 1980s, even the most distinguished British hospitals had long queues of patients waiting in surroundings of astounding shabbiness (creating what might be called an aesthetic barrier to utilization).[12] The BNHS had the longest waiting lists for surgical and other acute care procedures in the developed world.[13] This was true even for hip replacements and other interventions whose efficacy is incontrovertible. To quote a 1984 study by Henry Aaron and William Schwartz:

> One of the best known facts about the British health care system, both at home and abroad, is that the waiting lists for hip replacements are long and getting longer. In 1977 routine cases waited an average of thirteen to fourteen months and urgent cases an average of four months; barely concealed within these averages were extreme delays of up to five years, with even urgent cases waiting two or three years. Waiting lists grew 31 percent between 1977 and 1979.[14]

The top-down budgeting process and the devolution of rationalizing decisions to the regional and district level also biased the BNHS against diagnostic and therapeutic innovation. In the context of a tight, independently fixed global budget, funds for innovation tend to come at the expense of already established services. As a 1984 editorial in a leading British medical journal, *Lancet*, explained, regional and district allocation committees were always "paying Paul at the expense of robbing Peter."[15] If "Peter" was an innovative technology, it lacked the political advantages of incumbency and seldom garnered sufficient support to secure new funding—the budget process thus tended to perpetuate the medical status quo.

Not unnaturally, after four decades the British became international laggards in most areas of medical innovation. As they came to appreciate their status, they rationalized it in senses never intended by the founders of the BNHS. Thus, the British tended to eschew conventional measures of effectiveness (for example, preventing preventable morbidity or mortality such as end-stage renal disease, or ESRD), preferring instead to measure the provision of "services that most people use most of the time."[16] Administrators and consultants (that is, hospital-based attending physicians) took comfort from the works of British theorists like A. I. Cochrane and Thomas McKeown, who were skeptical about the impact of acute, emergency, and tertiary care interventions on health, and who insisted upon extremely high standards of proof before acknowledging the effectiveness of a medical innovation.[17] These theories legitimated Luddite attitudes, rationalized the perpetuation of the status quo, and provided those working within the financially strapped system with a justificatory rhetoric of demanding proven "value for money." They enabled the British to point with pride to the fact that they spent less of their gross domestic product on health care than did any other country in the Western world. These theories allowed them to argue that it is not they who are tightwads but the rest of the world that is spendthrift.

On a more personal level, consultants and specialists needed to rationalize the denial of known effective treatment to their patients. Aaron and Schwartz believe this led them to "rationalize" in the psychiatric sense of the term:

Resource limitations put doctors in a position that many of them find awkward. Trained to treat illness, they find they are unable to provide all the care from which their patients might derive benefit. . . . Wherever possible . . . [d]octors gradually redefine standards of care so that they can escape the constant recognition that financial limits compel them to do less than their best.

By various means physicians . . . try to make the denial of care seem routine or optimal. . . . The British nephrologist tells the family of a patient . . . that dialysis would be painful and burdensome and that the patient would be better off without it; or he tells the resident alien from a poor country that he should return home, to be among family and friends who speak the same language—where, as it happens, the patient will die because dialysis is unavailable. . . .

In each instance physicians are asserting that the treatment is *medically* optimal or very close to optimal, that the patients denied care or provided alternative forms of care because of budget limits lose essentially nothing of medical significance. For the undialyzed patient who dies, for the victim of angina who must bear pain . . . this view is unpersuasive. . . . But it enables doctors to avoid the painful realization that they are doing less than the best for the patient.[18]

Ultimately, rationalizing also meant limiting consumer-patient powers of protest. As early as 1950, general practitioners forced the erection of bureaucratic barriers that effectively denied patients the ability to change GPs.[19] In 1980, as the public began to realize that it was being denied effective treatment, patients petitioned the courts to redress the systematic underfunding of nonprimary care service— and the British court formally reneged on Bevin's promise of universalizing the best.[20] "It can not be supposed that the Secretary of State has to supply all the latest equipment [or] to provide all the kidney machines that are to be asked for, or . . . all the new developments, such as heart transplants, in every case where people would benefit from them."[21] The court's opinion unmasks rationalizing as rationing, and makes it clear that "health care for all" does not mean that the British people would receive all the health care that they "would benefit from."

IS NONMARKET RATIONING IN THE BNHS
JUST OR EQUITABLE?

Many commentators still look to the BNHS, or to its younger Canadian cousin, as a model for U.S. health care reform.[22] Contemporary British analysts, however, tend to be more circumspect. They recognize that their system never fulfilled its original ambitions, wryly remarking that it "universalized the adequate."[23] The argument here is that rationing within the BNHS is more morally problematic than is generally appreciated and ultimately stems from the fixation of its founders on monetary barriers to access.[24] Then, as today, many commentators saw money and markets as the root of all inequity in health care provision and tried to prohibit monetary barriers to access. By doing so, they also eliminated the "visibility" of market rationing, thereby violating formal constraints of justice more profoundly than the market. Sadly, the available data indicate that these formal violations have led to inequities—inequities that are unjust *even* according to the standards accepted by the founders of the BNHS.

In his influential 1971 book, *A Theory of Justice*, the philosopher John Rawls proposed formal conditions that any theory of just allocation must satisfy.[25] Although scholars have challenged other aspects of his theory, these criteria have been well received. Perhaps the most important of them is *publicity*, under which, to quote Rawls, "nothing is or need be hidden" about allocation decisions, because "everyone accepts and knows that others likewise accept the same principles," and knows that they apply to the social institution in question, and furthermore knows, or has access to, the reasons that the allocation is done in one way and not another.[26] Rawls sums up the need for such publicity as follows: "Publicity ensures, so far as the feasible design of institutions can allow, that free and equal persons are in a position to know and to accept the background social influences. . . . Being in this position is a precondition of freedom: it means that nothing is or need be hidden."[27]

Rationing within the BNHS violates Rawls's publicity condition. It is *invisible* in the sense that decisions "do not appear . . . as a *decision that had been made* . . . to deny . . . therapy."[28] Before the 1980s—when the Thatcher government publicized the extent to which the BNHS rationed coronary care, hip replacement, intensive care, kidney dialysis, neonatal intensive care, and a myriad of other acute and tertiary care interventions—the British public was almost entirely unaware that access to known effective treatments was rationed within the BNHS. This is not to deny that the BNHS budget was debated in Parliament; rather, it is to assert that the realities of denied medical care tended not to be understood, either by those debating the pounds and pence of the BNHS budget or by the public.

To elucidate the sense in which rationing in the pre-1980 BNHS can be considered "invisible," consider the practice of denying patients access to acute or tertiary care on the grounds of "old age" (that is, over fifty years old).[29] Physicians engaging in this practice were not applying a standard that, according to Rawls, "everyone accepts and knows that others likewise accept." To be sure, ethical theorists as distinguished as Daniel Callahan and Norman Daniels have argued cogently in favor of using chronological age to ration access to health care.[30] The British public, however, was never informed that when they passed age fifty their entitlement to acute and tertiary care would be diminished; nor have they ever formally accepted the principle of rationing access according to chronological age. Absent any public consensus, the physicians denying treatment to the middle-aged and elderly had little choice but "to tell lies to older patients, partly to make the patients more comfortable, and partly to make ourselves more comfortable. We have to say to them that their hearts are too dodgy to stand the strain on dialysis."[31] In effect, therefore, age rationing tended to be invisible to the patient, and, insofar as physicians lied to themselves, even to the rationing practitioners—hence it was also invisible to parliament and the public.

To someone of a pragmatic turn of mind, a few white lies to sugar-coat the realities of rationing are insufficient grounds for impeaching a system. Some commentators, most notably Guido Calabresi and Philip Bobbitt, argue that it is essential to hide so-called tragic choices from public view to "preserve the moral foundations of social cooperation."[32] (Henry Aaron echoes this sentiment at some points in his paper in this volume.) To these theorists, the criterion for judging the morality of the BNHS, or any other system of health care delivery, is essentially the New Testament test: "By their fruits ye shall know them." The moral question, for pragmatists, is not whether British clinicians lie, but whether the fruit of the system is sweet or bitter. Thus, pragmatists might indict the U.S. health care system, not on the grounds of some philosophical abstractions but because, as a matter of fact, in 1987, 47.8 million Americans lacked health insurance for at least one month, 24.5 million lacked it for the entire year, and one in five children was uninsured.[33] In short, moral pragmatists judge markets, or medicaid, or, returning to the immediate point, the BNHS not in terms of moral theories but in terms of the actual impact of the system on the population. To the pragmatist, unless one can adduce "real" evidence that invisible rationing leads to real suffering, charges of violating the publicity principle advanced by Rawls are entirely academic—in the most pejorative sense of the term.

The BNHS is able to ration invisibly because health care demand is mediated through professionals, and the BNHS has trained its professionals to conceptualize patient needs, *not* in terms of medically ideal treatments but in terms of treatments that give the patients their "fair share" of the resources available. The BNHS physician is thus trained to act as a gatekeeper as well as, and sometimes rather than, a health restorer. This strategy of cost containment has been effective and (until recently) noncontroversial. Yet, filtering patient needs through the subjective lens of physicians' perceptions of "fairness" also creates a potential for bias. Unfortunately, the best available data indicate that biases actually influence the allocation of acute and tertiary care services in the BNHS.

One bias that is ironic—in light of the Labour government's avowed intent of founding the BNHS as a vehicle for purging class biases from British society—is that against the lower and working classes. According to a recent study, the middle and upper classes "obtain a higher proportion of the resources of the health service than would be expected by chance, and a much higher proportion in relation to their needs when compared with others in the community."[34]

These biases appear to be an indirect result of the gatekeeper role required of BNHS physicians. For in playing this role, largely male, middle-class, young or early-middle-aged, white, nonimmigrant general practioners, consultants, and specialists are asked to allocate resources to a population of patients that is largely non-male, non-middle-class, above early-middle-age, and increasingly nonwhite and immigrant. The values of the gatekeeper and the kept are thus different. Even the most humane and democratically inclined of gatekeepers might be tempted, in such a context, to open and close the gate according to their own values, rather than the values of the patients they shepherd.

The BNHS's selection of a treatment modality for ESRD is a case in point. ESRD patients can be dialyzed either in their homes or in hospitals. Home dialysis, however, places a premium on education and self-discipline, which are values endorsed by the middle class. Hospital-based dialysis, in contrast, requires neither education nor self-discipline (and is the preferred mode amongst the working and lower classes in the United States). The BNHS opted, however, for home dialysis. Although the decision was rationalized in terms of "value for money," by opting for a modality acceptable in terms of their own values (but which is less than optimal for the working class), the clinicians of the BNHS inadvertently biased the allocation of ESRD treatments toward people like themselves and against the working classes.[35]

Implicit value biases that favor the upper and middle classes are inherent in the gatekeeper system and appear to be widespread in the BNHS. They are quite different from the covert, but nonetheless *explicit*, bias of the BNHS—such as the bias against patients over fifty. The difference is that implicit biases operate at a subconscious level, whereas explicit biases are at least occasionally recognized as "understood," if unstated, criteria that all gatekeepers use—that is, denying access because of age in the BNHS is "the done thing." All people in the system know that it is done—even though they are reticent to speak about it among themselves and conceal it from their patients.

Age, of course, sometimes serves as a prognostic indicator (that is, it may indicate the likelihood that an intervention will have a successful outcome). But it is important to appreciate that, according to internationally recognized standards, there is no prognostic or physiological reason to restrict dialysis (or admission to coronary care units, and so forth) to people under the age of fifty—although there are clear economic savings in doing so, because the over-fifty population has the greatest need of dialysis (and coronary care units, and so on). The inevitable effect of restricting access to life-sustaining interventions for patients over fifty is that they will die prematurely. To prevent such deaths for ESRD patients, the United States provides dialysis free of charge to everyone, regardless of age, under the Social Security Act.

By 1986 approximately one-third of the patients receiving dialysis in the United States were over sixty-five. More than 10 percent of the patients receiving dialysis in the United States are over seventy-five.

In contrast, "the United Kingdom treats almost none [of the over seventy-five] population at all."[36] The British provide kidney dialysis for men over fifty at about half the rate of such European countries as France, Germany, Italy, and Spain. Moreover, in those countries the number of patients per million (PMP) treated *increases* as the population ages—presumably in response to increased need. In Britain the number of men treated in the over-sixty-five population *decreases*—as a consequence of age-rationing—to between one-half and one-third of that in other European countries (some of which, by the way, have a lower per capita income than Britain).

The situation is even worse for women, especially for those over sixty-five, who are dialyzed at the extremely low rate of 22 PMP—that is, British women are dialyzed at a rate between one-third and almost one-fifth that of the rest of Europe.[37] The remarkably low dialysis rates for elderly women indicate that, in addition to being covertly "ageist," the BNHS is also "sexist"—that is, its gatekeepers' implicit gender biases appear to have exacerbated its explicit (albeit not publicly spoken) age biases. The largely male world of consultants and nephrologists who act as gatekeepers for ESRD treatment would appear to favor male exceptions to the rule of age rationing—seemingly finding it easier to deny dialysis to their female patients than to their male counterparts.

Age, class, and gender biases in the BNHS, whether implicit or explicit, are open to precisely the same moral objections that Labour made to market allocation of health care. The classic philosophical formulation of Labour's critique was penned by the philosopher Bernard Williams (at one time husband of the Labour minister, Shirley Williams) in his often quoted 1962 essay "The Idea of Equality."

> The proper ground for the distribution of medical care is ill health; this is a necessary truth. . . . [I]n very many societies, while ill health may work as a necessary condition of receiving treatment, it does not work as a sufficient condition, since treatment costs money and not all who are ill have the money; hence the provision of money becomes . . . an additional necessary condition for actually receiving the treatment. . . . [Thus] we have straightforwardly the situation of those whose needs are the same not receiving the same treatment, though needs are the grounds of treatment. This is an irrational state of affairs.[38]

Cutting through the philosophical jargon about "necessary condi-tions," the gist of Williams' argument is that, in the light of the aims of medicine, people with the same medical needs ought to receive the same medical treatment; it is inequitable, and "irrational," in the sense of being contrary to the aims of medicine, for them to receive different treatments.

Whatever one's assessment of Williams' argument (there are some classic critiques),[39] it should be evident that, insofar as it is valid, it also applies to age, gender, and social-class rationing. For, as Williams said, when these factors bias the allocation of treatment, "we have straightforwardly the situation of those whose needs are the same not receiving the same treatment." In sum, the very arguments that La-bour leveled against market rationing also apply to the nonmarket rationing mechanisms used by the BNHS.

There is also a real sense in which the invisibility of rationing in the BNHS leaves the British public—especially the working class, those over fifty, and women—worse off than they were under market ra-tioning. It is an often overlooked virtue of the market that the invis-ible hand has publicly recognizable, visible effects. To paraphrase an old folk song, "When living (or health care) is something that money can buy, the rich will live, and the poor will die." Before the BNHS, the knowledge that money is the passport to medical care (or, to speak the jargon of philosophers, a "necessary condition" for such care) gave the British working and middle classes a reason to organize privately to form so-called friendly societies and other forms of vol-untary and employer-provided health insurance. They also organized politically to ensure a measure of government-backed health insur-ance.[40] It also permitted the poor and their partisans and benefactors to develop a network of charity hospitals and clinics.

Invisible rationing, however, denies the public the power of re-sponse. Recall the political controversy that arose over the introduc-tion by the BNHS of drug, dentistry, and eyeglass fees in the 1950s. The controversy attests to the public virtue of visible rationing; that is, visibility allowed the public to act, either through protest, politics, or personal decision (such as buying insurance, seeking charitable aid, and so forth). The invisibility of the alternative mechanisms used by the BNHS since that time has denied the public these options. Only in the 1970s, when the extent of rationing became clearer to the British public, did it begin to take political action, to organize charities (providing support for kidney dialysis and other treatments),[41] and, most sensibly, to purchase supplemental health insurance.[42] Before this, the invisibility of the BNHS rationing rendered people powerless to control basic decisions affecting their lives—leaving those less favored by the BNHS more powerless than they would have been under a system of market rationing.

RELEVANCE OF THE BNHS TO THE UNITED STATES AND TO THE OREGON INITIATIVE

Reflection on the BNHS experience challenges several clichés that pass as conventional wisdom among American health care pundits. The first is that, except for the two "USAs"—the United States of America and the Union of South Africa—every nation in the industrialized world provides universal access to health care to its citizens. In truth, every health delivery system in the world *limits* access to health care, even—despite its motto of "free health care for all"—the BNHS. Moreover, although no American government ever promised to "universalize the best" as the British Labour government did on July 5, 1948, President Lyndon Johnson, when he signed titles 18 and 19 of amendments to the Social Security Act (more popularly known as medicare and medicaid) into law, on July 30, 1965, initiated programs designed to make health care accessible to all medically underserved Americans.

The American strategy was comparable in intent to, but different in methodology from, the British. Medicaid and medicare are "categorical" programs, in the sense that they target two specific "categories" of medically underserved populations—the elderly and the poor. The middle and upper classes, it was presumed, could either purchase their own health insurance or would have it provided by their employers. Thus, the intent of the U.S. categorical access and the British universal access initiatives was the same—to ensure unlimited access to health care for all.

Budgetary realities, however, ultimately eroded the actual extent of unlimited access in both the United Kingdom and the United States. After a surprisingly brief flirtation with the unrationed nonmarket provision of health care, both countries reneged on the commitment to unlimited access by instituting mechanisms of invisible rationing.

The mechanisms of disentitlement, however, are significantly different in the two countries. Britain places the power of disentitlement in the hands of gatekeeping physicians. In the United States, the fiction of unlimited entitlement tended to be preserved at the physician level, and disentitlements are achieved through bureaucracies of reimbursement. In Oregon, for example, eligibility for medicaid was set at 50 percent of the poverty level—those below this line received unlimited access to resources, those above the line, but still below the poverty level, received none. Title VI of the Social Security Amendments of 1983 is another example: it initiates a prospective payment system for hospitals (known as the diagnosis-related group, or DRG, system), which cleaves the relationship between the fees the government pays for services and the actual cost of the services paid for. More important, it develops an incentive structure encouraging hospital administrators to pressure physicians to expedite treatment—even at the risk of undertreatment and premature discharge.[43] An even more blatant example of the American system of bureaucratic disentitlement is the state of New York's practice of reimbursing a medicaid patient's initial office visit to a physician at the paltry rate of eight dollars—less than one-fifth of the actual cost. Private practice physicians cannot afford to provide services at such a substantial loss, and so, simply by setting a low reimbursement rate, New York effectively denies medicaid patients access to primary care, while shamelessly proclaiming that it provides an unparalleled system of health care for the poor.

In America, as in Britain, rationing tends to be "invisible" to the patient and often to the physician as well. Neither medicaid patients who are unable to find a private physician, nor medicare patients who are discharged early from a hospital, are in a position to perceive the mechanism that denies them access—they may not even realize they have been denied access. Nor, for that matter, are physicians in a position to see the patients who are discouraged from seeking access to primary care, or (except in extreme cases) those sent home early from the hospital. Thus, as in the United Kingdom, the abstruseness of the mechanisms of disentitlement disguise the realities of rationing both from those being rationed and from those legislating and administering the rationing—leaving the rhetoric of unlimited access untouched.

This leads us to the second cliché that passes as conventional wisdom in American health policy analysis—the view that *before* America experiments with rationing, it should first experiment with national health insurance. The truth about U.S. health care rationing is that it is really an artifact, not of the market but of a failed 1965 attempt to create a national health insurance program. The reality is that medicaid (and, increasingly, medicare), though formally committed to providing unlimited access to health care for certain categorically defined populations, has failed to do so not only in Oregon but in every state in continental America.[44] What is important to appreciate is that, as in the United Kingdom, the failure to replicate, in a nonmarket system, the three primary market functions of priority setting, resource generation, and "demand curtailment," or rationing, has led to shortfalls in funding and to invisible rationing. What the U.K. and U.S. experience shows is that the strategy of simply legislating access (whether categorical or universal)—the strategy that is still recommended by Sara Rosenbaum of the Children's Defense Fund (see her paper in this volume)—will not actually provide such access unless and until we develop explicit standards of rationing.

This introduces the third cliché that passes for conventional wisdom: the belief that rationalizing the U.S. health delivery system will eliminate the necessity of rationing. Here, for example, is what the political scientist, Lawrence Brown, says on the subject.

> Oregon's contribution is mainly to show that, at least today, in the United States, rationing is not a profound, but a spurious issue. . . . The United States should worry less about rationing and more about constructing a rational policy framework whose watchwords are budgeting, planning, regulation, and negotiation. If the polity declines to make these hard choices, rationing can not save it from itself. American policymakers have not earned the right to ration health care, and the very policies that would earn it the right would eliminate much of the urge to exercise it.[45]

Physicians for a National Health Plan offer a similar analysis,[46] which is echoed in this volume by Representative Sanders and several of the physician contributors, such as Anthony Tartaglia. The history of the BNHS, however, provides an almost definitive demonstration of the fallaciousness of this approach.

Budgeting or rationalizing and other administrative innovations yield at most a one-time cost savings—in the British case, even that achievement is dubious. Ultimately, without some systemic mechanism for financing the costs of medical innovation, demand will outstrip resources. The example of the BNHS (and our own experience with medicaid and medicare) shows that when this increased demand is experienced by a health delivery system operating under a mandate to provide unlimited access, budgeting or rationalizing almost inevitably translates into invisible rationing. The crisis of the medically unserved and underserved in both the United Kingdom and the United States is thus an artifact of a misguided belief in rationalization. Further attempts at budgeting or rationalization will only exacerbate the underlying problem. A permanent solution requires developing a mechanism to increase the supply of services to meet new demand, or to prioritize and curtail demand, or both—in other words, rationing.

REFLECTIVE COMMENTS ON THE OREGON INITIATIVE

A number of perceptive analysts (including Stephen Ayres and Norman Daniels) recognize the need for rationing but argue that it is best performed by individual physicians.[47] Four decades of microrationing by the physicians of the BNHS demonstrates, however, that microrationing, because it is invisible, is potentially discriminatory (in the case of the BNHS, against those over fifty, the working class, and women). It also corrupts the integrity of the patient-physician relationship, forcing physicians not only to lie to their patients but also to rationalize by refusing to recognize their patients' needs as needs. The moral health of all social institutions, and the psychological integrity of anyone involved in rationing, requires that the process be public at all three Rawlsean levels—that the principles of rationing be publicly recognized, that the public know they are being applied to medicine, and that reasons for the specific decisions be made known.

Henry Aaron and John La Puma are both concerned that explicit public rationing will be subject to political demagoguery, or will unduly infringe on the physician's autonomy and obligation to serve the patient, or both. These are reasonable concerns, as are those voiced

by La Puma and Robert Veatch about the details of the Oregon rationing system. I believe with Rawls, however, that publicity is not only a
"precondition of freedom" but a catalyst for reform. I am confident,
therefore, that if the Oregon rationing plan proves problematic in the
ways envisioned by Aaron, La Puma, and Veatch, the same open and
democratic processes that led to the initial design will rectify any
problems that emerge after it is implemented.

Norman Daniels, Bernard Sanders, and other commentators are
also apprehensive about the multitier nature of the Oregon initiative.
Their concern focuses, not unreasonably, on the fact that in the Oregon legislation explicit rationing applies primarily to medicaid recipients. What they fear is that, because most middle-class voters will not
be affected by the rationing scheme, they will, to paraphrase La Rochefoucauld's famous maxim, "have strength enough to endure the
misfortunes of others." The history of health care rationing, however,
challenges La Rochefoucauld's view of the public conscience. For the
truth of the matter is that neither the Americans nor the British have
had the fortitude to endure the misfortunes of others. Both have rationed stringently, but they needed to create elaborate rationaliza-
tions to hide their rationing decisions from themselves. The strategy
of the Oregon initiative rests on the presupposition that these ration-
alizations play an important role in the public psyche. Hence, by removing the reality-disguising fiction of fractions (for example, 50 percent of the poverty level), by making the suffering of others visible to
the legislature and to the public—so that all will know precisely what
they deny to others when they vote a certain budget—the initiative
will make it difficult for the public to endure the misfortunes of others. In the end, the Oregon Plan rests on the presumption that when
the public is faced with open, honest, visible decisions about health
care, it will do the decent thing.

From a moral and philosophical perspective, the Oregon initiative
is a watershed in the history of the nonmarket provision of health
care. For the first time, a funds-providing body has publicly admitted
the impossibility of providing unlimited access to health care, es-
chewed abstruse reality-disguising budgetary devices, and opted for
an allocation process that makes the realities of rationing explicit and
visible to all. For this reason, if for no other, the Oregon experiment
deserves to be tried. It may well prove to be the most significant event
in the public provision of health care since the "appointed day."

NOTES

1. For further details, see the papers by Michael Garland and Jean Thorne in this volume.

2. Quotation from Thomas Halper's *The Misfortunes of Others: End-Stage Renal Disease in the United Kingdom* (Cambridge University Press, 1989), p. 22.

3. Henry Aaron and Tristram Engelhardt, Jr., hold that markets do not ration resources. In his paper Aaron defines *rationing* as "the denial to people who have the means to pay for health care some services that promise medical benefit. By that definition, the denial of health care to those who are uninsured is not what I call rationing." For Engelhardt's statement see his paper in this volume. The political scientist Thomas Halper makes the same point more formally by defining rationing as a "means of resource allocation at below market price" (*Misfortunes of Others*, p. 149). See also M. D. Reagan, "Health Care Rationing: What Does It Mean?" *New England Journal of Medicine*, vol. 319 (October 27, 1988), pp. 1149–51.

4. See Robert Baker, I. Alan Fein, and Martin Strosberg, "The Intelligent Anaesthesiologist's Guide to the Language and Logic of Allocation," *Anesthesiology Clinics of North America*, vol. 9 (June 1991), p. 443.

5. Scholars who opt for the narrow usage have difficulty making these comparisons. For example, the economist-physician team of Henry Aaron and William Schwartz, who wrote a landmark comparative study of American and British health delivery systems, typically eschew the term *rationing* in the comparative passages in their text. Henry Aaron and William Schwartz, *The Painful Prescription: Rationing Hospital Care* (Brookings, 1984).

6. The report, written by Sir William Beveridge and published in November 1942—that is, in the middle of World War II—contained a broad vision of the welfare state. Its central theme was that "want was a needless scandal due to not taking the trouble to prevent it." Churchill's wartime coalition government not only published the report, which became an immediate best seller, but distributed a condensed version to troops in the field. The report was thus seen as the government's promise to the British people for a better society after the war ended. Its basic recommendations were adopted, with only some modifications, when the Labour party won power. In the Beveridge Report, the net cost of a British National Health Service was estimated at £170 million (from the general budget), which was approximately the sum actually allocated by the government. In the event, however, the actual net costs were almost double—on the order of £300 million during the 1940s.

7. Brian Watkin, *The National Health Service: The First Phase, 1948–1974 and After* (London: Allen and Unwin, 1978), p. 28.

8. Quoted in Rudolf Klein, *The Politics of the National Health Service* (London: Longman, 1983), pp. 33–34.

9. The resignation of Bevin and Harold Wilson over the principle of "no

financial barriers to access" split the Labour party. For further details see Watkin, *National Health Service*, pp. 28–29.

10. The initial cap was a net £400 million. Ibid., p. 28.

11. Harry Eckstein, *The English Health Service: Its Origins, Structure, and Achievements* (Harvard University Press, 1958), p. 172.

12. There are two sets of "Thatcher" reforms: the first was proposed by Sir Roy Griffiths, in *NHS Management Inquiry* (London: Department of Health and Social Services, 1983), and attempted to introduce managerial responsibility into the BNHS, as well as some competition into the provision of the domiciliary services (catering, laundry, and so forth). The reforms of 1987–90 attempted to introduce the "social market" or "internal markets" into the BNHS. For an overview of the latter reforms, I recommend two publications: Ray Robinson and Kenneth Judge, *Efficiency and the NHS: A Case for Internal Markets?* Health Unit Paper 2 (London: Institute for Economic Analysis, 1988); and Ray Robinson and others, *Health Finance: Assessing the Options* (London: Kings Fund Institute, 1988).

13. John Yates, *Why Are We Waiting? An Analysis of Hospital Waiting Lists* (Oxford University Press, 1987).

14. Aaron and Schwartz, *Painful Prescription*, p. 58.

15. Halper, *Misfortunes of Others*, p. 62.

16. Brian Abel-Smith, "Minimum Adequate Levels of Personal Health Care: History and Justification," *Millbank Memorial Fund Quarterly*, vol. 56 (Winter 1978), p. 19.

17. Archibald Cochrane, *Effectiveness and Efficiency* (London: Nuffield Provincial Hospitals Trust, 1972); and Thomas McKeown, *The Role of Medicine: Dream, Mirage or Nemesis?* (London: Nuffield Provincial Hospitals Trust, 1976).

18. Aaron and Schwartz, *Painful Prescription*, p. 101.

19. Richard M. Titmuss, "The National Health Service in England: Some Aspects of Structure," in Richard M. Titmuss, *Essays on the Welfare State* (Beacon Press, 1958), pp. 138–40.

20. In its first two sections, the National Health Service Act of 1946 embedded Bevin's promise to "universalize the best," which give the public an unlimited right to access to health care. To quote the act:

> 1.—(1) It shall be the duty of the Minister of Health . . . to promote the establishment . . . of a comprehensive health service designed to secure the improvement in the physical and mental healths of the people . . . and the prevention, diagnosis, and treatment of illness, and for that purpose to provide or secure the effective provision of services in accordance with the following provisions of this Act.
>
> (2) The services so provided shall be free of charge, except where any provision of this Act expressly provides for the making and recovery of charges.

The drafters of the Act, however, allowed a measure of prudence in article 2.

> 2.—As of the appointed day, it shall be the duty of the Minister to provide throughout England and Wales, *to such an extent as he considers necessary* to meet all reasonable requirements, accommodations, services of the following description. . . .

The courts ultimately interpreted the obligations of the BNHS in terms of the italicized section of article 2.

21. *Regina* v. *Secretary of State for Social Services,* ex parte Hincks et al. (1980), 123 SJ 436.

22. See, for example, "Norman Daniels, Why Saying No to Patients in the United States Is So Hard," *New England Journal of Medicine,* vol. 314 (May 22, 1986), pp. 1380–83; the paper by Bernard Sanders in this volume; and John Holahan and others, "An American Approach to Health System Reform," *Journal of the American Medical Association,* vol. 265 (May 15, 1991), pp. 2537–40.

23. Rudolf Klein, *Politics of the National Health Service,* p. 147.

24. See article 1, as quoted in note 20.

25. John Rawls, *A Theory of Justice* (Harvard University Press, 1971).

26. John Rawls, "Kantian Constructivism in Moral Theory: The Dewey Lectures 1980," *Journal of Philosophy,* vol. 77 (September 1980), p. 537.

27. Ibid., p. 539.

28. Leonard Fleck appears to have been the first philosopher to have the ingenuity to use the term *invisible* as an antonym for Rawls's concept of *publicity;* I have appropriated and expanded the meaning of this felicitous bit of jargon (by claiming that rationing can be invisible not only to those denied treatment but also to those denying treatment). I commend the reader to Fleck's thought-provoking essay on Health Maintenance Organizations: Leonard Fleck, "Justice, HMOs, and the Invisible Rationing of Health Care Resources," *Bioethics,* vol. 4 (April 1990), p. 100.

29. Aaron and Schwartz, *Painful Prescription,* pp. 34–37; and Halper, *Misfortunes of Others,* pp. 120–28.

30. Daniel Callahan, *Setting Limits: Medical Goals in an Aging Society* (Simon and Schuster, 1987); and Norman Daniels, *Am I My Parents' Keeper: An Essay on Justice between the Young and Old* (Oxford University Press, 1988).

31. Quoted in Halper, *Misfortunes of Others,* p. 134. See also Aaron and Schwartz, *Painful Prescription,* pp. 36–37.

32. Guido Calabresi and Philip Bobbit, *Tragic Choices* (Norton, 1978), p. 18.

33. Emily Friedman, "The Uninsured: From Dilemma to Crisis," *Journal of the American Medical Association,* vol. 265 (May 15, 1991), p. 2491.

34. Julian Le Grand, *The Strategy of Equality: Redistribution and the Social Services* (Cambridge University Press, 1989), p. 28. See also Julian Le Grand, "The Distribution of Public Expenditures in the Case of Health Care," *Economics,* vol. 45 (May 1978), pp. 125–42.

35. See Thomas Halper, *Misfortunes of Others*, p. 24.

36. Ibid., p. 23.

37. All figures on dialysis are from ibid., pp. 22–23.

38. Bernard Williams, "The Ideal of Equality," in Peter Laslett and Walter G. Runciman, eds., *Politics, Philosophy and Society II* (Oxford: Blackwell, 1962); reprinted in Bernard Williams, *Problems of the Self: Philosophical Papers, 1956–1962* (Cambridge University Press, 1973), pp. 240–41.

39. See, for example, Robert Nozick, *Anarchy, State and Utopia* (Basic Books, 1974).

40. From 1912 to 1949 the British also had a form of national health insurance. For details see Eckstein, *English Health Service*.

41. In the case of ESRD, two groups surfaced in the mid to late 1970s, the British Kidney Patient Association (BKPA) and an umbrella organization of local kidney patient groups, the National Federation of Kidney Patients Associations (NFKPA). The BKPA, led by Elizabeth Ward, is the most militant. She has been the least charitable about the BNHS's stoical fortitude at "endur[ing] the misfortunes of others." For details see Halper, *Misfortunes of Others*, pp. 75–81.

42. In the ten-year period 1979–89, the percentage of the British population with private health insurance doubled from 5 percent to 10 percent; half of this insurance is employer provided. Robinson and others, *Health Finance*, p. 22.

43. See Fleck, "Justice, HMOs," esp. pp. 102–03.

44. Friedman, "The Uninsured," p. 2492.

45. Lawrence Brown, "The National Politics of Oregon's Rationing Plan," *Health Affairs*, vol. 10 (Summer 1991), p. 50.

46. See Kevin Grumbaum and others, "Liberal Benefits, Conservative Spending: The Physicians for a National Health Plan Proposal," *Journal of the American Medical Association*, vol. 265 (May 15, 1991), pp. 2549–54.

47. See the papers by Ayres and Daniels in this volume. For a fuller statement, see Daniels, "Why Saying No . . . Is So Hard," p. 21.

Contributors

with their affiliations at the time of the conference

HENRY J. AARON, Senior fellow and director of the Economic Studies program, Brookings Institution

STEPHEN M. AYRES, Dean of the Medical College of Virginia, Virginia Commonwealth University

ROBERT BAKER, Professor and chairman of the Department of Philosophy, Union College

NORMAN DANIELS, Professor and chairman of the Department of Philosophy, Tufts University

H. TRISTRAM ENGELHARDT, JR. Professor at the Center for Ethics, Baylor College of Medicine

I. ALAN FEIN, Associate professor in the Department of Surgery, Albany Medical College

ARTHUR W. FLEMING, Professor and chairman of the Department of Surgery, Charles R. Drew University of Health and Science and King-Drew Medical Center, Los Angeles

MICHAEL J. GARLAND, Professor in the Department of Public Health and Preventive Medicine, Oregon Health Sciences University

EUGENE HARDIN, Vice chairman of the Department of Emergency Medicine, Charles R. Drew University of Health and Science and King-Drew Medical Center, Los Angeles

C. BOYD JAMES, Associate professor in the Department of Psychiatry, Charles R. Drew University of Health and Science and King-Drew Medical Center, Los Angeles

ROBERT M. KAPLAN, Professor in the Department of Community and Family Medicine, University of California at San Diego

JOHN LA PUMA, Director of the Center for Clinical Ethics, Lutheran General Hospital, Park Ridge, Illinois

E. HAAVI MORREIM, Associate professor in the Department of Human Values and Ethics, College of Medicine, Health Science Center, University of Tennessee at Memphis

GARY J. ORDOG, Associate professor in the Department of Emergency Medicine, Charles R. Drew University of Health and Science and King-Drew Medical Center, Los Angeles

SARA ROSENBAUM, Director of the Child Health Division of the Children's Defense Fund

BERNARD SANDERS, Member of the U.S. House of Representatives from the State of Vermont

WILLIAM SHOEMAKER, Chairman of the Department of Emergency Medicine, Charles R. Drew University of Health and Science and King-Drew Medical Center, Los Angeles

ROSALYN STERLING SCOTT, Associate professor in the Department of Surgery, Charles R. Drew University of Health and Science and King-Drew Medical Center, Los Angeles

MARTIN A. STROSBERG, Associate professor in the Graduate Management Institute, Union College

ANTHONY P. TARTAGLIA, Dean of Albany Medical College

JEAN I. THORNE, Director of the Medical Assistance Program for the State of Oregon

ROBERT M. VEATCH, Director of the Kennedy Institute of Ethics, Georgetown University

JONATHAN WASSERBERGER, Associate professor in the Department of Emergency Medicine, Charles R. Drew University of Health and Science and King-Drew Medical Center, Los Angeles

JOSHUA M. WIENER, Senior fellow in the Economic Studies program, Brookings Institution

RON L. WYDEN, Member of the U.S. House of Representatives from the State of Oregon

Conference Participants
with their affiliations at the time of the conference

Rosalie Abrams
Maryland Office on Aging

Stephanie Aldrich
Blue Cross/Blue Shield

Michael O. Allen
The Record

Signe Allen
*Union Labor Life Insurance
Company*

Ricardo Alonso-Zaldivar
Knight-Ridder Newspapers

Joseph Antos
*Health Care Financing
Administration*

Adrienne Appel
Internal Medicine News

Aurora Zappolo Argueta
*U.S. Department of Health and
Human Services*

Ross H. Arnett III
*Health Care Financing
Administration*

Thomas A. Ault
*Health Care Financing
Administration*

Jean Bandler
*New York University School of
Social Work*

Robert Barnes
Washington Post

Frank V. Booth
Buffalo General Hospital

Violet A. Boyer
Office of Senator Kent Conrad

Jack E. Bresch
Catholic Health Association

Gretchen Brown
Office of Senator Bob Kerrey

Jonathan Bynum
Union College

Letty Carpenter
*Health Care Financing
Administration*

Mary Brecht Carpenter
*National Commission to Prevent
Infant Mortality*

Howard Champion
Washington Hospital Center

Janet L. Chapin
*American College of Obstetricians
and Gynecologists*

Gary Christopherson
Gray Panthers

Steven B. Clauser
*Health Care Financing
Administration*

Howard Cohen
*House Committee on Energy and
Commerce*

Bente E. Cooney
*National Commission to Preserve
Social Security and Medicare*

David I. Cooper, Jr.
U.S. Department of Health and Human Services

Anthony M. Costrini, M.D.
Costrini, Meadows and Smith, P.C.

David J. Cullen
Massachusetts General Hospital

Julia Curry
Concern for Dying

William Custer
Employee Benefit Research Institute

Gerben Dejong
National Rehabilitation Hospital Research Center

James Dolph
Albany Medical College

Tim Eckels
Lewin/ICF

Erik Eckholm
New York Times

Jill Eden
Office of Technology Assessment

Marilyn Falik
MDS Associates

Sandra Fein
State University of New York at Albany

Steven Findlay
U.S. News and World Report

C. David Finley
St. Luke's/Roosevelt Hospital Center

Melvina Ford
Congressional Research Service

Julia R. Fortier
House Committee on Energy and Commerce

Peter D. Fox
Lewin/ICF

Michael G. Franc
Office of Representative William E. Dannemeyer

Joyce Frieden
Business and Health

William T. Friedewald
Metropolitan Life Insurance Company

Thomas C. Gabert
Wausau Medical Center, S.C.

Charles E. Gallagher
Hospital of the University of Pennsylvania

George M. Gill
ICI Pharmaceuticals Group

Karyn C. Gill
League of Women Voters of the U.S.

Marsha Gold
Group Health Association of America

Marian Gornick
Health Care Financing Administration

Thomas Grannemann
SysteMetrics

Daniel S. Greenberg
Science and Government Report

George D. Greenberg
U.S. Department of Health and Human Services

Darrel J. Grinstead
U.S. Department of Health and Human Services

Robert Griss
United Cerebral Palsy Association

Marcy Gross
U.S. Department of Health and Human Services

Thomas A. Gustafson
Health Care Financing Administration

Geri Hammond
National Association of Extension Home Economists, Inc.

Patrick B. Hazard
University of Tennessee

Tim Henderson
Office of Technology Assessment

Daniel L. Herr
Washington Hospital Center

Maria Hewitt
Office of Technology Assessment

David Holzman
Independent reporter

Thomas Hoyer
Health Care Financing Administration

Melody Hughson
House Committee on Energy and Commerce

Roger Hull
Union College

Judith Huntington
American Nurses Association

Allen Hyman
Columbia University

Lynn E. Jensen
American Medical Association

Richard Jensen
General Accounting Office

Tom Joe
Center for the Study of Social Policy

David Jonsen
University of Virginia Hospital

Ray Jordan
Pfizer, Inc.

David Kaufman
St. Vincent Hospital

Donald L. Kelley
Texas Department of Human Services

John H. Kelso
U.S. Department of Health and Human Services

Mary S. Kennesson
Health Care Financing Administration

Karin Janel Kimbrough
Office of Representative Donald Payne

Janet L. Kline
Congressional Research Service

Max E. Knickerbocker
HealthCare Facilities, Inc.

Richard Knox
Boston Globe

Bruce U. Kozlowski
Virginia Department of Medical Assistance Services

Shelah Leader
American College of Obstetricians and Gynecologists

Bonnie Lefkowitz
Bureau of Health Care Delivery and Assistance

Penelope Lemov
Governing magazine

Robert F. Leonard, Jr.
NYNEX

Margaret Levine
SUNY Downstate

Deborah Lewis-Idema
MDS Associates

Andrew Lipman
Union College

James D. Lubitz
*Health Care Financing
Administration*

Philip Lumb
Albany Medical College

Consuelo Mack
Wall Street Journal Report

Bruce K. MacLaury
Brookings Institution

Mary Faith Marshall
*University of Virginia Health
Sciences Center*

Nancy Mattison
Hoffman-LaRoche, Inc.

Gregory J. McGarry
Albany Medical Center

Jody McPhillips
Providence Journal

Rebecca R. Mendelson
*Office of Representative Alan B.
Mollohan*

Richard E. Merritt
*Intergovernmental Health Policy
Project*

Melissa A. Miccolo
*Dartmouth-Hitchcock Medical
Center*

Jessica Miller
Lewin/ICF

Vic Miller
*Federal Funds Information for
States*

Wilhelmine Miller
Georgetown University

Pamela Mittlestadt
American Nurses Association

Marilyn Moon
Urban Institute

Sara E. Morningstar
*Office of Representative Beverly
Byron*

Edmund C. Moy
*Health Care Financing
Administration*

Chris Murtaugh
*Agency for Health Policy and
Research*

Lisa Myrick
BNA's Medicare Report

Joe R. Neel
Physician's Weekly

Robert M. Nelson
Children's Hospital of Wisconsin

Jane Newman
Pfizer, Inc.

Daniel E. Nickelson
Cleveland Clinic Foundation

Margaret Ann Nolan
Maryland Office on Aging

Janet O'Keeffe
American Psychological Association

Victor Ostrowidzki
Hearst Newspaper

Alan Ota
The Oregonian

E. Veronica Pace
D.C. Office on Aging

B. Babu Paidipaty
St. Mary Hospital

Robert E. Patterson
Pennsylvania Blue Shield

Susan Pettey
*American Association of Homes for
the Aging*

Mary Plaska
National Association of Community Health Centers

Susan Polniaszek
United Seniors Health Cooperative

Elaine Power
Office of Technology Assessment

Gerald F. Radke
Pennsylvania Department of Public Welfare

Fedele F. Regan
League of Women Voters National Office

James R. Ricciuti
U.S. Department of Health and Human Services

Michael A. Rie
Harvard Medical School

Richard J. Riseberg
U.S. Public Health Service

Janet Rose
New Mexico State Agency on Aging

Elisabeth Rosenthal
New York Times

Cindy Rushton
Johns Hopkins Children's Center

Sarah Sa'adah
Office of Technology Assessment

Dallas L. Salisbury
Employee Benefit Research Institute

Elizabeth Sams
Washington Media Associates

Barbara Sander
Albany Medical College

Judith Sangl
Health Care Financing Administration

Yvonne Santa Anna
House Select Committee on Aging

Emily Santer
U.S. Department of Health and Human Services

Dawn Satterfield
Centers for Disease Control

Harry L. Savitt
Health Care Financing Administration

William Scanlon
Georgetown University

Catherine D. Schmitt
Blue Cross/Blue Shield of Michigan

David G. Schulke
Senate Special Committee on Aging

William E. Scott
Cooper Hospital/University Medical Center

Joseph P. Shapiro
U.S. News and World Report

Mildred B. Shapiro
New York Division of Medical Assistance

Daniel Shea
American Academy of Pediatrics

Gail E. Shearer
Consumers Union

Donald Shriber
House Energy and Commerce Committee

Andrew Smith
American Association of Retired Persons

Joseph L. Smith
Geisinger Medical Center

Patricia Smith
American Association of Retired Persons

Allen Spanier
Jewish General Hospital

Michael Specter
Washington Post

Arthur C. St. André
Washington Hospital Center

Susan Stasiewicz
St. Agnes Hospital

Mary Stuart
Maryland Department of Health and Mental Hygiene

Wayne Sulfridge
U.S. Department of Health and Human Services

Katherine Swartz
Urban Institute

Kathy Sykes
Office of Representative David Obey

Mary Takach
Office of Representative Joe Kennedy

Daniel Teres
Baystate Medical Center

Kenneth L. Toppell
Park Plaza Hospital

Sidney Trieger
Health Care Financing Administration

Joan F. Van Nostrand
National Center for Health Statistics

Lynn Wagner
Modern HealthCare

Edwin L. Walker
Missouri Division of Aging

Julie Walter
Union College

Julie H. Walton
Health Care Financing Administration

Dorothy Warner
Coopers and Lybrand

Caryn Weiss
St. Luke's Roosevelt Hospital Center

Marina Weiss
Senate Finance Committee

Steven C. White
American Speech-Language-Hearing Association

Dennis Williams
U.S. Department of Health and Human Services

T. Franklin Williams
National Institute on Aging

David P. Willis
U.S. Public Health Service

Angelique Wolf
Union College

Leah Wolfe
Office of Technology Assessment

Karl D. Yordy
Institute of Medicine